THE

BANTING

POCKET
GUIDE

THE
BANTING
POCKET
GUIDE

Prof. Tim Noakes
Bernadine Douglas
Bridgette Allan

PENGUIN BOOKS

Published by Penguin Books
an imprint of Penguin Random House South Africa (Pty) Ltd
Reg. No. 1953/000441/07
The Estuaries No. 4, Oxbow Crescent, Century Avenue, Century City, 7441
PO Box 1144, Cape Town, 8000, South Africa
www.penguinbooks.co.za

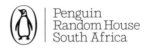

Penguin
Random House
South Africa

First published 2017
Reprinted in 2017, 2018 (twice) and 2019

5 7 9 10 8 6

PUBLISHER: Marlene Fryer
MANAGING EDITOR: Ronel Richter-Herbert
EDITOR: Bronwen Maynier
PROOFREADER: Ronel Richter-Herbert
COVER DESIGN: Monique Cleghorn
TEXT DESIGN: Ryan Africa
TYPESETTING: Monique van den Berg

Set in 10.5 pt on 14 pt Minion

Printed by **novus print**, a division of Novus Holdings

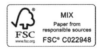

MIX
Paper from
responsible sources
FSC® C022948

ISBN 978 1 77609 155 3 (print)
ISBN 978 1 77609 156 0 (ePub)
ISBN 978 1 77609 168 3 (PDF)

Contents

Dedications

I would like to dedicate this book to my Creator; only He can give one the wisdom and knowledge to write a phenomenal book like this pocket guide. I would also like to dedicate this book to my mother, who has taught me so many things in life; most importantly, that one should always chase one's dreams and never, ever give up, no matter how hard life can sometimes be.

And lastly, to my two beautiful children: in between school, homework, meals and bath time they knew Mommy had to work on this book to finish it on time, and as young as they are, they understood perfectly.   – BERNADINE

To my immediate family, Ross, Anne, Belinda, Warwick, Ryan, Megs and Quintin for their ongoing encouragement and unconditional love. To Inben, my partner, best friend and fellow champion of the LCHF lifestyle, for his support and unwavering faith in my ability to meet deadlines. Also to Cara and Cody, my most beloved and loyal companions, who have enhanced my life immeasurably.

– BRIDGETTE

We would also like to thank The Noakes Foundation for their hard work in bringing world-class research to the table. With the creation of their Eat Better South Africa! project, they are making it possible for each and every South African to maintain a healthy lifestyle. A big thank you to Jayne Bullen, and a special thank you to the man who initiated this endeavour in South Africa, Prof. Tim Noakes.

— BERNADINE & BRIDGETTE

To my wife, Marilyn Anne, the most caring and intellegent being I have ever met, for a fabulous 50 years together. To our children, Travis and Candice, for being themselves and for their love and care for us and their children. And to the best legal team in the world: Attorney Adam Pike, Advocate (Dr) Ravin 'Rocky' Ramdass and Senior Counsel Michael van der Nest for their selfless support during my 'Banting for Babies' trial, when I, Marilyn and our children needed it the most. We can never repay the debt we owe you for your brilliance, your humanity and your generosity.   — TIM

We would also like to thank Penguin Random House, Marlene Fryer, Ronel Richter-Herbert and Surita Joubert for their hard work, dedication and team effort in helping us to bring you this pocket guide.

Introduction

Why is it that the Banting eating plan has attracted such a massive following in South Africa and, increasingly, around the world?

The simple answer is: because it works. And it works for reasons that we may not yet fully understand. But, most probably, because this is the single eating plan that best suits our unique human biology. Its key effects are (1) to reduce hunger, allowing us to effortlessly eat fewer calories and therefore lose weight without being perpetually hungry; and (2) to reduce our blood insulin levels, allowing us to burn the fat that we eat rather than store it, as happens in those who have high blood insulin levels because they eat high-carbohydrate diets.

While it is also true that no single diet will ever be ideal for every single human, the Banting eating plan ticks more boxes for more humans than perhaps any other. But most especially for those with insulin resistance (IR), type 2 diabetes mellitus (T2DM) and/or metabolic syndrome, which increasingly is becoming most of us. The latest projections suggest that at least 50 per cent of diverse populations across the globe have IR because they have already been diagnosed with T2DM or pre-diabetes.

Today it is estimated that 420 million people around the world have T2DM. Five million died of the disease in 2015; that's one person every six seconds. T2DM currently consumes up to 12 per cent of all the money spent on health care globally; in some countries, this share is up to 20 per cent. Projections for the future are even direr: by 2040, it is estimated that one in every 10 humans will be diabetic.

South Africans are among the worst-affected peoples. A recent study found that one in three Zulu-speaking males over 65 years living in Durban has T2DM. And it is perhaps even worse in Cape Town: another local study found that 28 per cent of a random sample of Capetonians have T2DM, which is equivalent to rates present in the 10 000 inhabitants of the Pacific Island state of Nauru, regarded as the nation with the world's highest rate of T2DM.

What makes these numbers truly disturbing is that the cause of T2DM is absolutely clear. It is a condition that occurred infrequently 100 years ago. Rates of T2DM took off in the late 1990s, exactly 20 years after the United States Department of Agriculture introduced novel dietary guidelines in 1977, now known as the 1977 US Dietary Guidelines for Americans (USDGA).

Those guidelines unwisely – because they were not based on any scientific evidence whatsoever – advised us to reduce the amount of fat that we eat and to increase substantially the proportion of carbohydrate, especially from cereals and grains, in our diet. The problem that should have been foreseen is that encouraging people with IR to eat less fat and more carbohydrate, regardless of source, will have only one outcome: rising rates of T2DM and other conditions linked to IR, including obesity, high blood pressure, gout, dementia and perhaps even cancer.

It follows that if we wish to reverse the global epidemic of obesity, T2DM, dementia and perhaps cancer, the solution is relatively simple: return to eating those foods that we ate in the 1960s before the 1977 dietary change that sparked the obesity/T2DM crisis.

Yet national governments and health-care systems across the globe seem oblivious to this fundamental truth. Instead we are reassured that T2DM is the inevitable consequence of being human in the 21st century; since it is an irreversible disease, we must simply accept reality. And if, as the popular story goes, we don't know what causes the disease, obviously we cannot prevent it. So for those who develop the condition: well, you have our medical sympathy, but it was probably your own fault that you developed T2DM in the first place. So we'll treat you as best we can. But we all know (although we won't admit it) that our treatment won't really make too much difference in the long run. In the end you are likely to become just another statistic, one of those deaths from T2DM every six seconds, month after month, year after year, decade after decade, forever more.

But some of us don't see it this way, so our message is quite different: if no one else is really interested in protecting our health, then the only option is for each of us to take care of ourselves.

This book therefore continues the tradition of South African authors driving the global Banting revolution by providing information that empowers those who wish to look after their own health by reverting to the traditional foods that we humans ate when we were last properly healthy, lean and non-diabetic, as most of us were in the 1960s.

So what is new in the world of Banting that makes us even more convinced that this eating plan is the solution for so much of the ill health that we see daily all around us and which, in the fullness of time, threatens to bankrupt global medical services and perhaps even the viability of certain nations?

1. BANTING WAS THE ORIGINAL DIET. IT CAN NEVER BE CALLED A 'FAD DIET'.

As described in *The Real Meal Revolution*, Banting was the original diet prescribed by William Harvey MD for his overweight patient, London undertaker Mr William Banting, in the 1860s. The diet was so successful that Banting described it in his iconic book *Letter on Corpulence: Addressed to the Public*, perhaps the very first 'modern' diet book ever written. The Banting diet was then taken to Germany and improved by a German cardiologist, Wilhelm Ebstein, in his book *Treatment of Corpulence*. From there the low-carbohydrate, high-fat Ebstein/Banting diet travelled to America, finding a home in perhaps the most famous medical textbook of all time, Sir William Osler's *Principles and Practices of Medicine*, published in 1892. Thus the Banting diet, as refined by Ebstein, became the first modern diet ever sanctioned and promoted by the leading physician of the day, Sir William Osler.

It follows, then, that the diets that have come after the Banting diet can reasonably be termed 'fad diets'. And the most faddish diet in history is the one that is the most promoted, the 'heart-healthy, prudent, balanced, in-moderation' diet that was unleashed on an unsuspecting world with the publication of the 1977 USDGA; the very diet that unleashed the tsunami of obesity and diabetes that began in 1980, three years after the publication of those evidence-free and predictably harmful guidelines.

2. WHAT DO THE MOST RECENT (2015) REVISIONS OF THE USDGA NOW PROMOTE AS A HEALTHY DIET?

The 1977 USDGA, which introduced the world to lipophobia – the fear of fat – were in retrospect perhaps the greatest single error in modern medicine. For one simple reason: not only did these guidelines NOT make us 'heart healthier', but by igniting the 1980 obesity/T2DM tsunami, they were also responsible for causing more ill health than perhaps all the pandemics that have swept the globe in recorded human history.

For we now know that there is no body of convincing evidence to prove that cholesterol – allegedly caused by eating a high-fat diet – causes heart disease, or indeed any other harm to the human body. The 'evidence' for that unproven relationship was advanced by compliant scientists at the behest of industries that stood to gain financially from the global adoption of this false theory.

We now know that IR, T2DM and metabolic syndrome are the conditions directly linked to heart disease. And ground-breaking new work published in the last year shows that by causing the condition of non-alcoholic fatty liver disease (NAFLD) in those eating high-carbohydrate diets, the insulin-resistant liver provides the direct pathway by which diet causes heart disease. And it is carbohydrates, not fats, that cause NAFLD and, hence, arterial disease leading to heart disease.

So by encouraging us all to eat more carbohydrates and to avoid fats, the evidence-free 1977 USDGA produced the T2DM/NAFLD epidemic, the key feature of which is widespread arterial disease through all our vital bodily organs. Destruction of these key arteries in our eyes, brains, hearts, kidneys and limbs, legs especially, leads to blindness, heart attacks, strokes, kidney failure and lower-limb amputations for peripheral gangrene. In short, the guidelines designed to protect our arteries from attack by cholesterol are the direct cause of the worst forms of arterial disease ever experienced by humans in our long history. And this attack is led by continuously raised blood glucose and insulin concentrations in those with IR who, out of ignorance, continue to eat high-carbohydrate diets.

Predictably, those who drafted the 1977 USDGA do not now wish to take any responsibility for the mayhem they released on the world. Instead, they have subtly revised their most recent 2015 guidelines to distance themselves from the error, without actually admitting it to anyone.

So, unknown to most, the 2015 version of the USDGA **no longer places any upper limit on the amount of fat** that humans can be advised to eat. They even propose that '[dietary] cholesterol is no longer a nutrient of concern'. What, I hear you ask? Why are these authorities not transparent in what they write? Why do they not simply admit that they got it wrong in 1977 and that humans should never have been told to limit the amount of fat they might choose to eat?

The good news is that the 2015 version of the USDGA is, with two exceptions that we'll look at now, entirely compatible with the Banting eating plan detailed in this book. But if you speak to most doctors, cardiologists especially, anywhere in the world, they are likely ignorant of these changes. So they will continue to tell you to avoid dietary cholesterol and to limit your fat intake by eating a low-fat diet, which unfortunately will cause T2DM, NAFLD and worsened arterial disease in those with IR.

But thanks to the 2015 version of the USDGA, you can quietly inform your medical advisors that, well, actually it's time to get current. The dietary advice has changed. You may now eat as much fat as you like, provided that it is in the form of 'healthy' fat.

The first of the two remaining errors in the 2015 version of the USDGA is that they continue to promote cereals and grains as a healthy source of 'nutrient-dense' carbohydrates when there is clear evidence that, compared to the foods of animals sources, promoted by our Banting diet, cereals and grains are nutrient poor. In addition, there is no hard scientific evidence that cereals and grains have any special health benefits. Instead, there is growing concern that the protein (gluten) contained in wheat, barley and rye may produce the leaky gut syndrome that is linked to a range of auto-immune medical diseases, as well as the more minor but annoying medical condition known as non-coeliac gluten sensitivity in those who are allergic to gluten.

So if there is no evidence that cereals and grains are healthy and some evidence that they might be actively harmful, why do they continue to receive such positive health messaging? Could it possibly be that the overproduction of grains in the US over the past decades has now produced a surplus for which there is no longer any spare storage capacity? Who is going to eat all those grains if it were ever to be announced that grains might not be as healthy as the 1977 USDGA presumed?

The second error is the promotion of polyunsaturated 'vegetable' oil as a healthy substitute for the wrongly accused but entirely healthy saturated fats from animals, fruits like avocados, and nuts like macadamias and coconuts. In fact, 'vegetable' oils like sunflower, safflower, canola and corn oil have nothing to do with vegetables. They are oils extracted from seeds by complex industrial processes that, as almost everyone with no financial reliance on the commercial success of these products agrees, render them highly undesirable for human consumption. Indeed, there is no evidence that 'vegetable' oils are healthy, but much to suggest that our increasing ill health since 1977 may also be linked to the huge global increase in our use of these highly artificial, fake foods.

3. WHY DO SO MANY HUMANS DEVELOP A RANGE OF APPARENTLY UNRELATED MEDICAL DISEASES WHEN THEY INGEST HIGH-CARBOHYDRATE DIETS FOR MANY DECADES?

To appreciate which foods are best for our bodies, we need to understand some quite fundamental features of how our bodies process different foods, especially carbohydrates, and how this leads to ill health in those with IR.

There is one feature of human biology that has seemingly been ignored by biologists but which shows, in one easy lesson, why humans are not designed to consume large amounts of carbohydrate frequently. When humans ingest carbohydrate – it doesn't matter whether it is a low-glycaemic (complex) or high-glycaemic (simple) carbohydrate – we break it down into its basic constituent, glucose. But here is the surprise. **The total amount of free glucose in the healthy human body at any time is only five grams, the equivalent of two small packets of sugar of the**

kind that we liberally add to our teas and coffees with gay abandon. These five grams of free glucose exists in the five litres of blood that constitute our bloodstreams. So, when we eat carbohydrates, the digested glucose that is added to our blood must be quickly stored in our livers and muscles or used as a fuel by our bodies. Otherwise it will cause damage to many body tissues. Failure to keep the blood content at five grams (in five litres) causes T2DM. I, like all the other 420 million diabetics around the world, have T2DM because my bloodstream contains not five grams of glucose, but six grams. That is the tiny difference between robust health and T2DM. On such small differences does the health of the world depend.

The body has learnt to use the hormone insulin as an emergency mechanism to drive the glucose out of the bloodstream into the muscles and liver and so to protect the body from the detrimental effects of high circulating blood glucose concentrations. But like all emergency solutions, this short-term answer comes with long-term consequences:

- weight gain, since insulin is the fat-building hormone that also prevents the use of stored body fat, turning us into carbohydrate-, not fat-, burning animals;
- arterial damage leading to all the dread complications we see in those with T2DM;
- increased body fat around the internal abdominal organs, including within the liver (NAFLD);
- high blood pressure;
- gout;
- generalised whole-body inflammation;
- dysfunction of the mitochondria in many body organs (mitochondria are the cellular structures that provide all our energy); and
- impaired exercise performance.

But worse, the more insulin we secrete (or inject, if we are unfortunate enough to be prescribed insulin as the treatment for our T2DM), the more IR we become. This is because our tissues become increasingly more insulin resistant as they are exposed to more and more insulin on a daily basis in those with IR eating high-carbohydrate diets. In the end, the system simply fails and we have the condition of T2DM and all its manifest complications.

So we now know that it is these repeated spikes of insulin and glucose, experienced every few hours from birth to death in our modern carbohydrate-laden food environment, that are the principal cause of our tragically increasing levels of ill health.

But the good news is that, since we now know the enemy, we can find a solution. Which is simply to eat only as many carbohydrates each day as our individual bodies can tolerate. And to eat much less frequently than the three to six times a day we are currently advised.

This book once more shows us how all this can be achieved.

Perhaps we should make it as simple as possible. Why don't we return to the way we ate in the 1960s, when most humans were lean and non-diabetic?

Or is that really too simple to be a realistic solution?

4. IF INSULIN RESISTANCE, NOT CHOLESTEROL, IS THE KEY DRIVER OF OUR ILL HEALTH, WHICH BLOOD TESTS SHOULD WE BE USING TO GAUGE OUR LEVELS OF IR AND PREDICT OUR FUTURE HEALTH?

One of the key drivers of our ill health is the false idea that our blood cholesterol value is the ultimate test for predicting our future health. When I entered medical school in 1969, we were taught by cardiac experts such as Professor Christiaan Barnard – who performed the world's first successful human heart transplant – that a normal blood cholesterol value is 7.5 mmol/L. Today we are warned that any cholesterol value above 5.0 mmol/L is a warning that we are in imminent danger of suffering a heart attack.

This change has happened for one reason: those companies selling cholesterol-lowering drugs (statins) wish to have as many humans across the globe eligible (and advised) to use their product. So they have generated two key beliefs about cholesterol that almost everyone accepts as the incontrovertible truth: (1) it is essential to know our cholesterol 'numbers'; and (2) if we wish to live a long and disease-free life, we need to keep our blood cholesterol level below 5 mmol/L. For we all 'know' that the instant our blood cholesterol value exceeds 5 mmol/L, our only hope for a long and disease-free existence is to lower that value by taking statin drugs and eating a low-fat diet.

The result of all this is that since blood cholesterol concentrations naturally rise with age – probably for a very good reason, namely that this rise keeps us healthier as we age – there will come a time when almost everyone will be told they need to take statins. And to eat a low-fat, high-carbohydrate diet.

And if elevated insulin and blood glucose concentrations are the real cause of arterial disease, the result of measuring everyone's blood cholesterol concentrations – which will be above 5 mmol/L in many of us – will be that the most likely advice that most of us with IR or T2DM will receive is: eat a high-carbohydrate, low-fat diet and take a statin drug. Which is about the worst advice anyone with IR or T2DM can ever receive.

So to make sure that we receive the proper dietary advice, it is important that we each understand which are the best blood measures of our degree of IR and whether or not we are likely to develop T2DM. Table 1 below lists the blood values, blood pressures and body mass indices that provide the best information to answer these questions.

Blood parameter	Insulin sensitive	Borderline	Insulin resistant/ T2DM
HbA1c (glycated haemoglobin) %	4.5	5.5	>6.0
Gamma-glutamyl transpeptidase (GGT) activity (U/L)	<45	>45	>100
Fasting insulin concentration (mIU/L)	<2.0	2.0–10.0	>10.0
Fasting glucose concentration (mmol/L)	<5.0	>5.5	>6.5
Fasting triglycerides (mmol/L)	0.5	1.0–1.5	>2.0
HDL-cholesterol concentration (mmol/L)	1.6	1.4	1.2
Fasting total cholesterol concentration (mmol/L)	Of no value in determining extent of insulin resistance. Minimal value for predicting risk of future heart attack.		
Fasting LDL-cholesterol concentration (mmol/L)	Of no value in determining extent of insulin resistance. Minimal value for predicting risk of future heart attack.		
Blood pressure (mm/Hg)	<120/80	140/90– 150/95	>160/100
Body mass index (kg/m^2)	<24	24–28	>28

Table 1: Blood values, blood pressures and body mass indices indicating different levels of insulin resistance

Perhaps the best overall marker of IR is the value for glycated haemoglobin (HbA1c). This is a measure of a person's average blood glucose level over three months. The value arises from the ability of glucose to bind to proteins, causing a change in their structure and function. The most prevalent protein in blood is haemoglobin, so glucose will bind to that protein in proportion to the average glucose level in the blood (during the lifetime of those red blood cells), giving us the HbA1c value. The table shows the values that are found in those who are insulin sensitive, those who are borderline IR and those who are IR or have T2DM.

The key point is that the change from insulin sensitive with an HbA1c of 4.5 per cent to T2DM with a value of 6.5 per cent **does not occur overnight**. Rather, it takes years or even decades to go from being insulin sensitive to developing T2DM. This means that by simply knowing your own HbA1c value and those of your family members, you can very easily prevent the development of T2DM and its serious implications by reducing the amount of carbohydrate that you include in your diet.

My advice is that everyone should have their HbA1c measured, and not cholesterol, since the cholesterol value tells us nothing about our levels of IR and little about our risk for future heart attack (see Table 1). Once your HbA1c value exceeds 5.5 per cent, it is time to start reducing your carbohydrate intake to below 100 grams per day. Those with higher HbA1c values will need to eat even less carbohydrate, preferably closer to 25 grams per day.

If we were all to follow this advice, the T2DM epidemic would be stopped in its tracks.

The blood gamma-glutamyl transpeptidase (GGT) activity is a measure of the extent to which NAFLD has developed. Any value greater than 45 U/L means that you are eating too much carbohydrate, indicating the need to reduce your intake to prevent the serious complications of NAFLD.

Fasting glucose and insulin values are usually considered together, but there is an important difference. When fasting insulin rises to the values shown in Table 1, it is the first sign that you may be developing IR. Initially this will keep the fasting blood glucose within the normal range, but ultimately the IR in the liver will progress to the point at which liver glucose production rises and blood glucose levels also begin to rise. Thus it is more important to measure fasting insulin than fasting glucose.

Similarly, if you were to have the standard test for T2DM, the glucose tolerance test (GTT), the more important marker is the blood insulin response to glucose ingestion, not the glucose response itself. This is because the diagnosis of IR will be missed in those who secrete an excess of insulin but who are still sufficiently sensitive to that excess insulin to be able to maintain their blood glucose levels within the normal range.

Fasting triglyceride and HDL-cholesterol concentrations are also excellent markers of IR. Fasting triglyceride values rise and HDL-cholesterol values fall with increasing levels of IR. A fasting blood triglyceride value below 0.5 mmol/L is a sign of robust metabolic health.

Finally, blood pressure and body mass index rise with increasing levels of IR combined with higher carbohydrate intakes. Indeed, one of the first effects of a low-carbohydrate diet in those with IR is a rapid drop in blood pressure. Unfortunately, few doctors treating patients with high blood pressure ever ask their patients what they are eating. But the simple change to a low-carbohydrate diet may be all that many with hypertension need to 'reverse' their elevated blood pressures.

CONCLUSION

When I began my personal Banting experiment on 12 December 2010, I had no idea what I would discover. Perhaps the most important lesson I have learnt in the past six years is that what we eat is the single most important determinant of our long-term health. But this is not something that is widely appreciated.

We, the authors, trust that this book will help you understand what you need to eat to be healthy and vigorous, and live long lives.

Good luck as you implement these ideas and enjoy the remarkable benefits of eating the way for which we humans were designed.

PROFESSOR TIM NOAKES OMS, MBCHB, MD, DSC, PHD
(HC), FACSM, (HON) FFSEM (UK), (HON) FFSEM (IRE)
EMERITUS PROFESSOR
NOVEMBER 2016

PART 1

WHAT IS BANTING?

FOR THE READER WHO IS NEW TO BANTING

In the context of this book, 'Banting' is the word we use when referring to a low-carbohydrate, high-fat (LCHF) lifestyle. The Banting lifestyle advocates:

- a diet high in healthy fats and low in carbohydrates ('carbs');
- eating only real, healthy and fresh foods;
- following a nutritionally dense diet comprising meat, fish, eggs, nuts, healthy fats, and a variety of vegetables and fruit; and
- eliminating additives, chemicals, preservatives and other harmful ingredients.

Many of you wanting to embrace this lifestyle are overwhelmed by all the information available on social media and the internet. We are here to help you get started on this journey. You need to remember that there is no such thing as a one-size-fits-all lifestyle or diet. Each of us is unique and our nutritional needs must be treated as such.

WHAT BANTING IS NOT

Banting or LCHF is a LOW-carb, not NO-carb, way of eating.
    While we know that humans have no need to eat carbohydrates

to be healthy and energetic, we do not advocate the complete elimination of carbohydrates from the diet. The recommended level of carbohydrate consumption varies from person to person and depends on the individual's metabolic condition.

Banting is not vegetable, fibre and fruit free

Starchy vegetables high in carbs are not encouraged in large quantities. Banters are encouraged to eat a good variety of healthy, whole vegetables, primarily those that grow above the ground. The vegetables we eat on a low-carb diet are full of fibre, so essentially this should be seen as a high-fibre diet. Fruit is not encouraged for people who are metabolically ill, such as diabetics, because fruits are usually high in natural sugars. But this does not exclude even these individuals from eating whole fruit from time to time.

Banting is not a high-protein diet

Some people assume that this is a high-protein diet. It's not. It's a moderate-protein diet.

Banting is not a fat feast

Remember, if you eat too much of anything, you will gain weight. The worst advice you can give someone complaining about not losing weight is to tell them to increase their fat intake, and specifically by adding fat bombs and bulletproof coffees. Fat is extremely calorie dense, and fat-filled foods and fat-loaded drinks do not, in our opinion, have a place in a weight-loss programme, unless they increase your satiety, reduce your hunger and so help you to eat less without hunger.

Banting is not dangerous

Ketogenic (very low-carb, high-fat) diets have been used since the 1920s to treat illnesses such as epilepsy, and no harmful effects have resulted from a long-term ketogenic diet.

Banting is not a quick fix

Banting is NOT a diet, it is NOT a fad and it is definitely NOT a short cut to weight loss. It is a shift from how you are currently eating to a new way of living; in short, it is a lifestyle change.

WHO CAN BENEFIT FROM BANTING?

There is no debate among nutrition experts that everybody can benefit from removing processed foods, added sugars, refined carbohydrates and junk from their diets, but they don't all agree that we should all be eating low-carb diets. Indeed, it is not necessary for everybody to limit carbs substantially. There are people who tolerate a high-carbohydrate intake (of course, here we are referring to carbohydrates from whole-food sources).

It is important to mention here that slim is not necessarily healthy. It is quite easy for people to be metabolically unhealthy or to suffer the detrimental effects of a poor diet without being overweight. A low-carb diet is not just for those who need to slim down; it is very effective for correcting a number of health issues.

Studies have repeatedly shown that a diet low in carbohydrates and high in healthy fats comes out tops for the treatment of obesity, diabetes and metabolic syndrome, and for the correction of unhealthy cholesterol. The question is, then, are there any people who should be excluded from Banting?

Essentially, no.

This is not a one-size-fits-all eating plan. The level of carbohydrate intake can be adapted to the individual, and for those who are concerned about the consumption of too much saturated fat, there is the alternative of using monounsaturated fats like extra-virgin olive oil.

If you have any health concerns, it is always advisable to be guided by a Banting-friendly health-care professional before you commence a new eating plan.

PART 2

WHY DO WE GET FAT?

Conventional wisdom tells us that we get fat because we either eat too much food or exercise too little. The problem with this over-simplified explanation is that it does not tell us *how* we get fat.

What causes this fat accumulation, what regulates it, and how can we manage or control it?

The hormone insulin puts fatty acids into fat cells, so you could say that insulin drives fat storage. When insulin levels in our bodies are chronically elevated, fat accumulates in our fat cells. When insulin levels drop, fatty acids escape from our fat cells and our fat deposits shrink.

What drives insulin production?

The answer: two macronutrients – carbohydrates and protein.

Carbohydrates and proteins are what we call insulinogenic, i.e. they stimulate the production of insulin. The more carbohydrates you eat, the higher your insulin levels will be. And because carbohydrates have no satisfying properties – they do not make us less hungry; in contrast, they stimulate hunger – you end up eating more of them. The problem is that every time you eat those carbohydrates, your insulin levels go up and more and more fat enters your fat cells instead of leaving them.

The other driver of insulin is protein. If you consume too much protein, and especially those that have a higher insulinogenic effect, such as whey protein and milk, your insulin levels will rise. But if you consume too little protein, protein synthesis will not occur properly and the small amount you did consume will become insufficient to sustain your muscle mass.

Quantity of food

Many new Banters mistakenly think that Banting is an 'eat as much as you like' lifestyle or that they can eat freely from the green list. This is untrue. The LCHF/Banting lifestyle is about eating when you are hungry and eating until you are satisfied. Banting is a diet high in fats, moderate in proteins and low in carbohydrates. You will need to make sure that your protein intake per day is as close to spot-on as possible; that you lower your carbohydrate intake, but you do not exclude carbohydrates completely because, if you do, you will miss out on nutrient-dense vegetables; and, finally, that you accept that fat is not your enemy and never was. Fat can be eaten in greater amounts, BUT, as with everything, there is a limit to the amount of fat you should be eating depending on where you are in your weight-loss journey.

Quality of food

Know that the food you choose to eat will determine your weight-loss success. Note that if you suffer from a metabolic disease,* you should only eat from the green list. If you're one of the lucky ones and don't have a metabolic disease or are more carb tolerant than most, then you can eat from both the green and orange lists. But take note that when we talk about orange foods, we are really only referring to vegetables and berries. If you want to eat any of the

---

* Metabolic disease or syndrome is a collection of five of the following medical conditions: abdominal (central) obesity, elevated blood pressure, elevated fasting plasma glucose, high serum triglycerides, and low high-density lipoprotein (HDL) levels.

other sugary fruits, then rather see them as sweet treats to be eaten once in a blue moon.

WHAT ARE MACRONUTRIENTS?

Macronutrients are the nutrients that we require in our diet in large (macro) amounts to supply us with energy (fuel); to provide us with other essential nutrients like vitamins, minerals and amino acids (micronutrients); and to make us feel full (satiated). There are three major macronutrients that the human body needs in order to function properly: fats, proteins and carbohydrates. Each has a different role in the Banting lifestyle. Most of the foods you are going to eat when Banting contain at least two of the three macronutrients. For example, an egg contains about 6 grams of protein and 5 grams of fat. So, you cannot assume that when we say consume x amount of protein, that the protein will only come from the meat that you eat. You will find protein in vegetables, dairy, nuts and seeds, to name but a few. Similarly, carbohydrates are not only found in grains and cereals. They are spread all over the conventional food pyramid, in vegetables, fruits, dairy, nuts, seeds and even some meats!

The role of fats in Banting

- Fat is there to supply us with energy, with enough fuel to get us through the day with ease.
- When we eat a diet higher in fat, we fill up quicker and can go longer between meals.
- Fat adds flavour to our foods. Without fat, food tastes horrible. Have you ever noticed when you look at the label on a low-fat yoghurt product that while the fat value is low, the sugar content of the product is extremely high? This is because fat gives flavour to products; remove the fat and you instantly remove the flavour.

The role of proteins in Banting

- Protein is at the centre when it comes to the three macronutrients.
- It is crucial to eat exactly the right amount of protein when on this diet. Once you know what your protein intake should be, you can work out your fats and carbohydrates from there.
- Proteins require 'extensive mechanisms to digest, metabolise and eliminate' and lead to 'high satiety to avoid excess intake'.[*]
- Benefits of higher-protein, reduced-carb diets include increased weight loss, the protection of skeletal muscle, a reduction in body fat, increased thermogenesis (the production of heat in the human body), increased satiety and enhanced regulation of blood glucose levels.
- Protein is also responsible for the growth and repair of our tissues and cells.
- Protein is responsible for providing us with the building blocks of life: amino acids. Meat-protein sources contain all the essential amino acids that are absolutely vital for our various biological processes.

The role of carbohydrates in Banting

- Carbohydrates can be divided into three groups: simple carbohydrates, which are sweet and are the short-chain carbohydrates found in our food; long-chain starches, which get broken down into glucose in the digestive system; and fibre, which cannot be digested by our bodies, but which the bacteria in our gut use to maintain our digestive health.
- When we consume carbohydrates, the enzymes in our intestine converts these carbs to glucose. Some of the digestive glucose is sent to our muscles to be used for energy or storage, to our

---

[*] Presentation by Dr Donald K. Layman at the 13th Annual Nutrition Forum, 2013, available at https://www.youtube.com/watch?v=4KlLmxPDTuQ (last accessed September 2015).

brains and other organs to be used as fuel, or is converted to fat and stored in our fat cells for later use under the action of the hormone insulin.

- There is only so much carbohydrate that each of us can use or store as carbohydrate. So if you consume more than your body can metabolise, the rest will be stored as fat (once the muscle and liver glucose stores are filled). Because carbs provide us with no satisfaction, it's not long before we reach for them again. Once again the body takes what it needs for energy, and then stores the rest. This process will just continue like a bad song stuck on repeat unless we limit the amount of carbs we consume to give our body a chance to use our stored fats.

- Although Banting is a low-carb diet, carbohydrates are still extremely important to the lifestyle. Carbohydrates in the form of vegetables as per the green and orange lists are important to maintain a healthy lifestyle, purely because vegetables provide us with loads of fibre and also some essential nutrients, such as vitamins.

- Most of the carbohydrates you eat from now on will come from vegetables and a few other foods on the green list.

- Other carbohydrates like rice, pasta and refined grains are of little nutritional value (other than providing unnecessary energy) and should be avoided.

HOW MUCH IS ENOUGH?

Too much or too little fat

In reality, 'high fat' does not give you permission to go overboard on fat. What it really means is that you should be eating more healthy fats, specifically a combination of saturated and unsaturated fats, and that your total fat consumption per day in macronutrient value should be higher than your protein and carb consumption.

- Almost all the foods we consume contain plenty of fat. Everything from protein-rich foods like meats and dairy to fruits such as avocados and olives contain fat.
- A person with a very high body fat percentage naturally has enough fat stores and ideally should first burn the stored fat before consuming more.
- Giving someone with a high body fat percentage more fat means that his or her body will burn the fats he or she is eating before it will burn the stored body fat, resulting in a fat-loss stall.
- The greater a person's weight, the bigger their body fat percentage and the less fat they need to eat initially, when they start Banting.
- A smaller person or someone who doesn't have so much weight to lose can increase their fat intake to provide them with enough energy to get through the day.
- The bottom line: the more weight you lose, the more fat you can consume.
- A lifestyle high in unhealthy carbs and high in unhealthy fats will lead to weight gain – this is a scientifically proven fact.
- Remember, the key to Banting is to eat enough fat (and protein) to reduce your hunger and allow you to eat less – and so to lose weight.

Too much or too little protein

How much is too much when it comes to protein?
- The amount of protein you need to eat will depend on your goal – whether you want to lose weight or build muscle (in the case of bodybuilders) – your age, your level of physical activity, etc.
- Eating too much protein can result in your body converting any excess protein into glucose, and this can result in fat storage.
- In his blog Optimising Nutrition, Managing Insulin, Marty Kendall explains: 'High levels of protein will generate insulin which will reduce fat metabolism (i.e. lower levels of ketones).

If the pancreas is struggling to supply enough insulin to maintain blood sugars in those with marked insulin resistance, then the insulin load from protein will make it harder for your pancreas to keep up and achieve optimal blood sugars. If you are trying to lose weight, then excess insulin will also promote fat storage.'*

- Too little protein can also be problematic, as it can cause our health and body composition to suffer, leading to muscle loss.
- If we don't consume the right amount of macronutrient protein during each meal, protein synthesis will not happen optimally and the small amount of protein that we have consumed will not maintain our body muscle mass.
- This is why it's so important to eat the right amount of protein per meal, and why you need to try, at least, to get the value for this macronutrient spot-on.

Too many or too few carbohydrates

Is too much carbohydrate bad for you? The short answer is 'yes and no'. 'Yes' if you have a metabolic disease such as type 2 diabetes, in which case too many carbohydrates are very bad for your health because they cause you to oversecrete insulin. You need to remember that it is insulin – not carbohydrates – that is the key problem. Carbohydrates cause the oversecretion of insulin (hyperinsulinaemia), but it is the excess insulin that damages our bodies. At the end of the day, we are all unique and what may seem like few carbs for one person will be a lot for another. Once again, what works for one won't necessarily work for another.

- If you eat high carb and high fat, your body will first use up the carbs and only then use the fats. And, like the other macronu-

---

* Marty Kendall, 'Why we get fat and what to do about it V2', 22 June 2015, available at https://optimisingnutrition.wordpress.com/2015/06/22/why-we-get-fat-and-what-to-do -about-it-v2/ (last accessed September 2015).

trients, your body will use what it needs of the carbs for energy and store the rest.

- The bottom line is that a high-carb, high-fat lifestyle is by far the unhealthiest and most fattening.
- Carbohydrate intolerance is thought to be genetic, but worsens with age on a high-carb diet.
- When we eat carbohydrates, they convert to glucose in the body under the action of enzymes in our intestines.
- The glucose that cannot be used immediately as fuel or stored in the muscles and liver is converted to fat. In people who are insulin sensitive, carbohydrates are metabolised well. But those whose cells do not respond readily to insulin, because they are insulin resistant, are unable either to store or use carbohydrates to a normal extent. Instead, they must store any excess as fat.

PART 3

PREPARATION

Mental preparedness is extremely important when embarking on any new diet or way of life. We see so many people looking for ways to 'cheat' or substitute from day one, and this is not the way forward.

The essentials

- In order to reclaim your health or ideal weight, you need to leave old eating habits behind.
- You must commit to Banting properly from the start. It may be hard in the beginning, and sugar and carb withdrawal is no fun, but within a couple of weeks your newfound energy and lack of hunger will be well worth the effort.
- Cutting out addictive foods little by little is no way to end an addiction – it simply prolongs it. Going 'cold turkey' is by far the quickest way. For most people the side effects are not significant and only last a few days.
- Identify habits that you need to change – for example, stopping at the corner café on the way to work for a coffee and pastry. Rather keep great coffee at work so that you can make yourself a cup when you get there. Normally grab fast food at lunch time? Once again, plan ahead and pack a healthy lunch to take to work with you.
- Choosing the right time to begin is also important. Adopting a

new regime during a stressful period may not be the best idea, and many find starting a new way of eating during the holidays almost impossible. Identify a couple of relatively stress-free weeks to get into your new lifestyle, but be realistic and don't find endless excuses not to begin.

· Plan your meals for the week and then go shopping. Always remember, planning ahead is essential. One of the biggest pitfalls when starting on a new eating plan is a lack of planning.

Sort out the kitchen

Once you've decided to Bant, it is a good idea to take a few days to prepare properly. This includes cleaning out the kitchen, planning your first week of meals and shopping for the right foods.

· There is no point hanging onto foods that are not part of Banting 'just in case'. Removing temptation will make it much easier to stay on the rails.

· If you feel that throwing away food is wasteful, then donate what you are no longer going to eat.

· Be ruthless. Don't hold back on getting rid of any foods or ingredients that do not appear on the green list. You may find that your grocery cupboard looks really bare, but you will not need these foods at all.

· Eliminating processed foods can be a huge shift and not having the correct foods at home will result in frustration and could tempt you to throw in the towel.

· If you are living with others who are not Banting, try to keep those items that you can't have out of sight. Banting is not a deprivation diet, and because the food is really wholesome and tasty, it won't be long before the rest of your household comes on board.

Once you have cleared out your kitchen of red-list foods, it's time to stock up on the ingredients that you will need. There are a few essentials that every Banter should have:

- The fats that you use for cooking (coconut oil, butter, ghee, extra-virgin olive oil).
- Herbs, pure spices, fresh meat and fresh vegetables.

Standard swap-out list

Below is a swap-out list to help you replace any unhealthy foods you may have in your pantry and fridge with healthier, Banting alternatives. Add to your shopping list those items that appeal to you.

Cooking	
Clear out	*Replace with*
Sunflower oil Canola oil Spray and Cook Margarine	Coconut oil Butter (salted, plain or ghee) Lard Tallow (beef or mutton) Fat (duck, chicken, pork) Macadamia oil (low heat only) Bacon drippings
Baking	
Clear out	*Replace with*
Cake flour Bran flour Barley flour Cornflour Rice flour Soy flour	Almond flour Coconut flour Flaxseed flour Heba flour
Meat	
Clear out	*Replace with*
Processed meat like polony and viennas Processed cold meats Marinated meat	Real, fresh fatty meats (game, poultry, fish, etc.) Cured pastrami, salami and chorizo Organ meats (offal)
Dairy	
Clear out	*Use instead*
Processed cheeses (normally individually wrapped) Low-fat or reduced-fat cheese Low-fat or reduced-fat milk Canned cream	Real, fresh hard and soft cheese Full-fat cheese Full-cream milk, coconut milk, natural almond milk and sour milk (amasi) Fresh cream, coconut cream and sour cream

Vegetables	
Clear out	*Use instead*
Peas, corn, legumes, parsnips, peanuts and potatoes (regular)	Green-list fresh vegetables

Porridge/cereals	
Clear out	*Use instead*
Commercial porridge or cereal	Chia-seed porridge (see page 94) Coconut almond porridge (see page 94) Banting breakfast granola (see page 98) Heba porridge (see page 95) Heba pap (see page 95)

Spreads	
Clear out	*Use instead*
Commercial cheese spread Jams and jelly Peanut butter	Almond nut butter Macadamia nut butter Tahini/sesame butter

Sides	
Clear out	*Use instead*
Rice Potato mash Pastas	Cauli rice (see page 124) Cauli mash (see page 125) Zucchini/baby marrow pasta (also known as zoodles)

Salad dressings and sauces	
Clear out	*Use instead*
Commercial salad dressings Commercial mayonnaise Commercial tomato sauce Commercial chutney Commercial cheese/pepper/mushroom sauce	Avocado oil, extra-virgin olive oil, macadamia nut oil or Banting salad dressing (see page 129) Banting mayonnaise (see page 129) Banting tomato sauce (see page 130) Banting cheeky chutney (see page 131) Banting sauces (see pages 129 to 134)

Set goals

- Set a short-term as well as a long-term weight-loss goal. Often long-term goals can look a little overwhelming, so smaller immediate goals can help to keep you motivated. Every small immediate goal you meet will take you closer to your long-term goal.

- Visualising your goal is a good way to stay motivated. This is not necessarily just about dropping a clothing size. You may think about being able to fit comfortably into an airplane seat, for example. As you set your goals, visualise them and stay focused on one at a time.

- Another great way to stay inspired is to reward yourself as you reach each goal. This doesn't mean devouring a chocolate bar after a week of correct eating, but treating yourself in a fun, positive, *healthy* way.
- With each goal reached, increase the reward. So a pedicure for the first goal and perhaps a massage for the second. Write down the reward in your journal next to each goal.
- With positive thoughts, you are more likely to succeed than by punishing yourself when things don't go so well. Place a few positive and motivating quotes around the house where you can see them, such as on your bedroom mirror or on the fridge door.

Get support
- Enlist the support of trusted family members or friends and don't tell people who may try to sabotage your efforts.
- Finding someone to join you on your weight-loss programme may make meeting your goals easier.
- Online communities are also helpful for giving you the ongoing support you need and answering any questions you may have. On days that you feel like throwing in the towel, an online community can be a great place to find support.
- Some people find that broadcasting their weight-loss efforts to others in their social circles helps with accountability. As you reach your goals, pop them on your Facebook page or tweet your success.
- Remember that all change involves some stress, so give yourself a couple of weeks to adjust.
- Put off social events and try to avoid stressful situations, especially if you have been an emotional eater.
- Focus on the successful areas of your life and how good your

accomplishments made you feel. Think of how you achieved those successes and duplicate that behaviour in your weight-loss endeavour.

MEAL PLANNING

Counting calories and weighing and measuring food was never the intention of the Banting lifestyle, but we have found that for some people, keeping track of their intake is important when starting out. Below are two approaches to determining how much you should be eating for weight loss.

Tool 1: The simple way

If you feel you can carry on with Banting and lose weight without having to weigh and measure your food, then this approach is for you.

Fats

- Cook and fry all your meals in fat such as butter, and drizzle olive oil over your salads.
- A little bit of cream in your coffee should be fine if you are not sensitive to dairy.
- Raw nuts provide plenty of fat, as do fruits like avocados.
- Eat fattier cuts of meat and aim for protein-rich foods that are high in omega-3 fatty acids, such as marine seafood.
- Chia seeds are also rich in fat and are a good cereal substitute.
- If you follow this general advice, your fat macronutrient value will be higher than your protein value, which is what we are aiming for.
- It is difficult to recommend a gram value here, as it will depend on each individual's current percentage of stored fat.

Proteins

- Work on a 100–150 gram portion of cooked protein (meat or seafood) per meal.
- One portion contains 20–30 grams of net/macro protein, giving you a total of 60–90 grams of net/macro protein per day.
- Bear in mind that it has been shown that per-meal consumption of protein is more important than overall daily intake.[*]
- In order to ensure protein synthesis, the body requires 2.5–3 grams of the amino acid leucine. This amount of leucine is found in 20–30 grams net protein from meat and dairy sources.
- If you cannot make up your total protein requirements through the meat you consume, you can make up the balance with dairy products like cheese and cream. You can make up the balance of your protein by including nuts, seeds and vegetables in your meals.

Carbohydrates

- Aim to eat 25–50 grams of net carbs per day.
- If you have a metabolic disease or are sensitive to carbohydrates, eating less than 25 grams net per day will be more beneficial.
- Get your carbs from vegetables at every meal.

Tool 2: Personal calculation of ratios

In a clinic consultation, we will typically calculate your daily macro-nutrient ratio. Based on information you supply, we will tell you that you can eat x grams of fat, x grams of protein and x grams of carbs. Here is what we take into account when we do a ratio report:

- History and current health status.
- Lean body mass (LBM) and current body fat percentage.

---

[*] D.K. Layman, '*Dietary Guidelines* should reflect new understandings about adult protein needs', *Nutrition & Metabolism*, 6(12), March 2009, doi: 10.1186/1743-7075-6-12.

- Current weight, age, height and gender.
- Activity levels.

Feel free to contact us for an online or face-to-face consultation: our contact details are on page 171 at the back of the book.

Choosing your meal plan

We have saved you some time by giving you four meal plans (see Part 7) to choose from. They are well balanced and contain enough vegetables to fulfil your daily nutrient requirements, and we have worked hard to ensure that the macronutrient value for protein falls within the recommended range of 20–50 grams net per meal. Note that each meal plan is generically designed and is meant as more of a guideline to help you learn portion control. If you don't have success on a meal plan, we suggest you give one of the other plans a try or contact us to assist you further with a personalised meal plan.

BASIC RULES OF BANTING

1. Banting is about eating when hungry and stopping when satisfied.
2. Eat clean, fresh, real food. Real food rots and has a very short shelf life. Do not eat processed or pre-packaged foods.
3. Make sure that you include fats, proteins and carbs in all your meals, whether you are eating three meals a day or only two. Meals must be nutrient dense and well balanced.
4. Do not eat more than three meals a day; there is no rule dictating which time of the day you should eat or that you have to eat all three meals.
5. Do not have sweeteners in your coffee or tea; go cold turkey if you want to see results.
6. Drink water throughout the day, but only when you are thirsty.

We recommend between two and three litres of water per day, but you know your body and how much you can handle. Coffee and tea count towards your daily water intake.

7. Make sure you are getting enough vitamins and minerals. If you experience energy loss in the beginning, you may supplement.

8. Do not drink any fizzy drinks, fruit juices or 'slimming' drinks, not even if they claim to be sugar free. They all contain artificial sweeteners and additives that can have a negative effect on your health and weight.

9. Do not snack between meals unless you are really hungry. Snacking between meals can lead to weight gain. If you are hungry, drink a glass of water – sometimes thirst is registered by the brain as hunger. Ask yourself why you snack – is it because you are bored, emotional, stressed or really hungry?

10. What works for you may not necessarily work for others. We are all unique. Don't blame Banting if someone else's meal plan doesn't work for you. If you want to try a meal plan, start with one of the four we provide in Part 7 of this book. The meal plans are well balanced and show the macronutrient break-down for each day.

11. Don't keep adding fats. There are more than enough fats in the foods you will be eating.

12. Eat vegetables. They make up most of your allowed carbo-hydrates for the day.

13. Avoid counting calories. In the beginning you want to consume less fat to give your body the opportunity to use its stored fat for fuel. If you follow calorie recommendations, you may end up eating too much fat.

14. If you need to count anything, count macronutrients (proteins, carbs and fats), but pay particular attention to keeping your carb count low.

CONSCIENTIOUS SHOPPING

In order to help you make informed decisions about the types of food you buy, here we take a look at terms such as 'organic', 'grass-fed' and 'grain-fed'.

Organic

- Organic foods are produced using organic farming methods. While standards differ worldwide, organic farming in general features cultural, biological and mechanical practices that foster the cycling of resources, promote ecological balance and conserve biodiversity.
- Synthetic pesticides and chemical fertilisers are not allowed.
- Organic foods are also not subjected to irradiation, industrial solvents or synthetic food additives.
- According to one study, '[o]rganic crops, on average, have higher concentrations of antioxidants, lower concentrations of Cd (the toxic metal cadmium) and a lower incidence of pesticide residues than the non-organic comparators across regions and production seasons'.[*]
- Organic foods are more expensive, so the choice is often budget-related.
- At the end of the day, irrespective of whether the vegetables are organic or not, they add variety, interest and bulk to meals.

Grass fed vs grain fed

- Grass-fed beef comes from cattle that have eaten only grass and forage (like hay or silage) from weaning to harvest.
- Some producers put the animals on grain for the last 90–160 days before slaughter. During this time the levels of important

---

[*] Marcin Barański, *et al*, 'Higher antioxidant and lower cadmium concentrations and lower incidence of pesticide residues in organically grown crops: A systematic literature review and meta-analyses', *British Journal of Nutrition*, 112(5), September 2014: 794–811.

nutrients like conjugated linoleic acid (CLA) and omega-3 decrease dramatically in the animal's tissues.

- Grass-fed beef has a distinct grass flavour; keep this in mind when cooking it. You may also notice that the fat from grass-finished beef has a yellowish appearance.
- Grain-fed beef comes from cattle (sometimes referred to as 'corn-fed', 'grain-fed' or 'corn-finished') that are typically fattened on maize, soy and other types of feed for several months before slaughter. As a high-starch, high-energy food, corn decreases the time it takes to fatten the cattle and increases carcass yield. Some corn-fed cattle are fattened in concentrated animal-feeding operations known as feedlots.
- Ruminants like beef cattle are not designed to eat grains. Grain-fed cattle are unhealthy and require antibiotic treatments to reach their goal weights. It is grains (carbohydrates) that fatten cattle, and the same applies to humans. This has been known for centuries.
- Grass-fed beef is obviously better in quality and nutrient value, but once again your decision will likely come down to budget.

READING FOOD LABELS

Reading food labels is important, but learning how to read them is crucial if you want to ensure that you are buying a good-quality, low-carb product. Below is an example of a typical food label. We will discuss what each listed item means and what you need to look out for. We will also give you warning tips to help you make informed decisions.

Typical nutrition information			
Serving size = 40 g			
	Per 100 g	Per serving	% NRV
Energy (kJ)	1 505 kJ	602 kJ	

Protein	9.4 g	3.8 g	
Glycaemic carbohydrate Of which sugars	67 g 1.1 g	27 g 0.4 g	10%
Total fat Of which saturated fat Polyunsaturated fat Trans fat	3.4 g 0.5 g 1.7 g 1.2 g	1.4 g 0.2 g 0.7 g 0.5 g	18% 15%
Cholesterol	15 mg	30 mg	10%
Dietary fibre	10.2 g	4.1 g	0%
Sodium	392 mg	157 mg	20%
Potassium	350 mg	700 mg	20%
Vitamin A	18 µg	36 µg	4%

Serving size

When reading food labels, it is important to ask what the serving size is, and is what I'm about to consume the equivalent of that serving size. Foods are listed in either grams (for solids) or millilitres (for liquids), and will include the nutritional information for 100 grams/millilitres of the product as well as for a serving size – in this example, 40 grams. Most serving sizes are really small. In a perfect world we'd keep to the serving size, but in reality most of us will consume more. So don't be fooled when the carbohydrates per serving size appear low; chances are you will be eating more than the recommended serving size.

Energy

Kilojoules (kJ) are units of energy. Calories and kilojoules are often used interchangeably on labels: 1 calorie = 4.12 kilojoules. Luckily on Banting we don't count calories or kilojoules.

Protein

Protein is listed in macronutrient gram value and can be given as a percentage of the national reference value (NRV). If you want to know how much protein you should eat, refer back to the section on meal planning.

Carbohydrates

According to new food-label regulations, carbohydrates are supposed to be listed as 'glycaemic carbohydrates', also known as net carbohydrates. This is the carbohydrate quantity available for metabolism and which will produce an insulin response. Fibre cannot be metabolised by the body and therefore does not count. Some old food labels, however, still have carbohydrates listed as 'total carbohydrates', which means the fibre content was not deducted from the total. Keep this in mind when reading labels. If the label refers to total carbohydrates, look for the fibre value and deduct this amount from the total carb amount to get the glycaemic (net) carbohydrate amount.

Sugar is listed underneath carbohydrates because it is a form of carbohydrate. Also note that should the product contain any starch, the starch will make up part of the glycaemic carbohydrate as well.

Total fat and cholesterol

Fats are usually broken down into the different types, namely saturated, unsaturated and sometimes trans fats. Buy full-fat products, and avoid products that are low-fat, fat free or reduced fat. Stay clear of products that contain trans fats, sometimes listed as hydrogenated vegetable oil in the ingredients. Cholesterol is another type of fat contained in certain foods. Note that cholesterol in foods does not raise the blood cholesterol concentration.

Dietary fibre

Dietary fibre sometimes makes up part of the total carbohydrates. See the section on carbohydrates above for more information on this.

Vitamins and minerals

If the product contains any vitamins or minerals, they will also be listed on the food label. Vitamins and minerals can either be found naturally in the product or are added. Nutrients are listed in their relevant unit of measurement, and indicated as a percentage of their NRV, which is the daily amount of the nutrient that most people need.

Other important information
Ingredients
The ingredients list is even more important than the nutritional value of the product. Before you look at the net carb value, you should look at the ingredients. If the product has more than two to three ingredients, then it's likely processed and will contain all sorts of unhealthy additives. Avoid the product if the list starts with sugar, refined grains, hydrogenated oils or a word that you cannot pronounce.

Allergy warning
If the product contains any ingredients to which some people may have an allergic reaction, the label should say so. This may include terms such as: 'this product was made in a factory that uses tree nuts'. It may be labelled 'lactose free' or 'gluten free'. Preservatives such as MSG (monosodium glutamate) and tartrazine can also cause allergic reactions and must be displayed on the label.

Organic
If a product claims to be organic, it must adhere to the regulations set out in the Agricultural Product Standards Act and be certified organic. This means that the product must come from farms, processors or importers who are registered with and approved by organic certification bodies.

Health claims
No food or drink label may claim that the product can treat, prevent or cure a disease or medical condition, for example 'calcium

enriched to prevent osteoporosis'. It's against the law to make any medical claims.

Warning tips for reading labels

Even though new label regulations for South African products have come into effect, there are still many wrongly labelled products out there. Always keep an eye open for deceptive or ambiguous claims. Here are some examples:

- 'Diabetic' products like diabetic sugars and jams that claim to be safe for diabetics, but which contain artificial sugars that are harmful, or fructose, which is as bad as sugar. The only sugar substitutes you can trust are xylitol, stevia and erythritol. So, unless the product contains these and nothing else, it's not diabetic friendly. But remember, we do not advocate the use of any sugar substitutes.
- Vitamin-enhanced drinks like vitamin waters that read 'contains antioxidants' or 'vitamins'. These types of drinks are just a fad and contain more sugar than anything else, as well as many other unhealthy ingredients.
- If the label reads 'light/lite', 'low-calorie' or 'low-fat', it means that the product was either watered down or fat was removed and replaced with sugar.
- 'Multigrain' and 'made with whole grain' mean the product con-tains either more of one type of grain or very little whole grain. Look at the first few ingredients to see if whole grain is listed.
- Fizzy drinks. These contain nearly eight teaspoons of sugar per 350-millilitre can. Manufacturers usually express the sugar con-tent in grams, so that the drink appears to have less sugar. Zero and lite fizzy drinks may not have natural sugar, but they still contain sugar substitutes, which we do not recommend.
- Fruit juices, even those that claim to be 'sugar free'. They might not have any added sugar, but they contain fructose, which is still a constituent of sugar.

- Similarly, products that say 'no added sugar'. They might not have added any more sugar to the product, but the product may still contain sugar naturally.
- Products with endorsements from health foundations. Certain margarines in particular are advertised as 'heart healthy', but if you look at the ingredients, you will see that they contain vegetable oils. Stay far, far away!
- Anything containing additives like preservatives, flavourings, etc., or listing a million E numbers (codes for natural and artificial food additives). They might look like food, they might even taste a little bit like food, but that long list of ingredients equals fake food.
- If the label has the name or address of some chemical laboratory, rather leave it. This is a clear warning that the product is highly processed.
- Be wary if the label reads 'zero trans fat'. All it means is that the product per serving must contain less than 0.5 grams of trans fat, but we now know that serving sizes are not reliable. You must not eat any trans fats.
- Manufacturers use many names to disguise the presence of sugar in their products. Look at the Ingredients List in Part 8 for the different names given to different types of sugar. Should you find more than two to three of these sugars listed on the label, avoid the product.
- Real foods hardly need labels. You should be able to tell what the ingredients are just by looking at the food.

PRODUCTS: THE GOOD, THE BAD AND THE UGLY

Real: not imitation or artificial; genuine
Food: something that nourishes, sustains or supplies

One of the focal points of Banting is to eat *real* food. One of the major drivers of the obesity and diabetes epidemics is the consumption of processed foods. With Banting on the rise, we have seen an influx of so-called low-carb, guilt-free products. A healthy and effective low-carb diet, however, needs to be based on the consumption of *real* food. We therefore need to be vigilant and informed so that we do not fall back into the processed pit.

- Real food is as close to its natural and original state as possible. It is recognisable.
- Pumpkin looks like pumpkin, meat looks like fresh animal flesh, fish looks and smells like fish.
- Real food includes fish, meat, vegetables, nuts, seeds and fruit. It does not come packaged with a long shelf life. It was recently alive, either on the tree or in the ground or out to pasture.
- Real food is not made in factories or laboratories, and it certainly does not come with a list of chemical additives and preservatives. Of course, for convenience's sake, some foods are now packaged, like olive oils, milk and butter, as well as some fresh ingredients.

Ingredients

One sure way for a Banter to trip up is to start indulging in baked goods that require 'Banting-friendly' ingredients. Some of these ingredients are useful and can be a part of Banting, but you need to learn to differentiate between what is a real-food ingredient and what is not.

- Real-food ingredients are derived from whole foods. These include nut flours that are ground directly from nuts (you can do this at home with a coffee grinder) and do not contain any fillers, sugar or preservatives. The most common nut flours are almond flour and coconut flour. Also acceptable are hazelnut flour and macadamia nut flour. Pure nut butters, such as almond butter and macadamia butter, are also 'legal'.
- Only *pure* spices are allowed. By pure spice we mean a spice derived from dried seeds, fruit, roots, bark or vegetables. The

name of the spice will correspond to the name of the seed or plant, e.g. cinnamon, nutmeg and ginger. BBQ is *not* a plant or seed.

- Always check the label. We are frequently asked if blends of certain spices can be used, and invariably these blends are full of MSG, fillers, preservatives and often sugar.
- Some spice blends, like a masala for curries, are acceptable, but once again be sure that there are no additives. Many spice stores do not package their spices, which are therefore not labelled, often giving the impression that the spices are pure. So always be sure to ask.

Low-carb products

A 'product' is an article or substance that is manufactured or refined for sale. Right away this falls out of the category of real food. You should therefore automatically stay away from any 'product' claiming to be low-carb or Banting friendly.

We tell you that reading labels is so important, but what do you do when food companies put false labels on their products? Fraudulent labelling can have serious health consequences, and it's the reason we are trying so hard to get you to buy and prepare your own real food. Many products labelled 'Banting-diet friendly' are definitely not. We have seen coconut sugar, peanut butter, rice flour and even quinoa labelled this way, none of which are acceptable ingredients for a Banting lifestyle.

Canned foods

Certain canned foods are acceptable. While fresh is always better, it's not always practical or possible.

- If you do purchase canned foods, make sure they are not loaded with sugar and soaked in vegetable oils and preservatives.
- Canned fish like tuna is fine as long as it is the one in brine or olive oil, and not vegetable oil or tomato sauce.

- Some canned tomato brands are fine, but be careful of added sugar. The same applies to tomato purées.
- If you drink instant coffee, check that the contents are pure coffee beans only. You will be shocked at just how many additives there are in some instant coffees, including sugar.
- Many people ask about coconut milk and coconut cream. You need to take care here. Commercial brands generally have additives to prevent the water and coconut oil from separating, and may have sulphites added to keep the product white longer. Incredibly, some also have added sugar. Organic ranges are available, but these are very expensive and not easy to come by. If you are a purist, you may want to steer clear of commercial brands.

Diet bars and shakes

- Optimal health is important for losing weight and maintaining weight loss. So, continuing to make poor food choices and substituting real food with processed bars is not wise.
- Over the years diet companies have been cashing in on our lazy eating habits. What starts as a healthy whole-food diet often becomes bastardised as greedy corporates seek to profit off desperate people looking for the quickest route to weight loss. These products are *not* an appropriate part of a healthy diet or lifestyle.
- Many of these products are not really even low-carb. They catch you out by listing the quantity of carbs per serving. One little snack bar may have 8.5 grams of carbs, but check per 100 grams and you'll find that it has a whopping 23 grams of carbs.
- Take a look at the ingredients in a typical snack bar: soy protein isolate, calcium carbonate, oat flour, oat fibre, glycerine, polydextrose (synthesised from glucose and sorbitol, and one of several newfangled fibre additives), chocolate-flavoured chips (made from maltitol and chocolate liquor), cocoa butter, soy lecithin, palm kernel, palm oil, sunflower oil, soybeans, artificial flavours,

dicalcium phosphate, salt, sucralose and sodium metabisulfite. Then there's the dark-chocolate-*flavoured* coating (it's not real chocolate!), titanium dioxide colour, yellow 5 lake, blue 2 lake, red 40 lake, etc.

- Diet shakes are no better. Add to this unhealthy line-up a host of other chemicals and laboratory-manufactured additives. Most shakes have a high soy content, and while some are low-carb, the majority are not, containing on average 13 grams of carbs per serving and sometimes a whopping 9 grams of sugar! That's more than two teaspoons of sugar per serving.

- Don't fall for bars and shakes that claim to support Banting. *Nothing* that sits in a container on a shop shelf with a list of additives, soy and an expiry date sometime in the distant future can be part of the Banting lifestyle.

Sugar-free sweets

Sugar-free sweets are just as bad. Many people who change to the Banting lifestyle are battling with sugar addiction and eating sweets in any form will only perpetuate the addiction. Of further concern is that many of these so-called sugar-free or low-carb sweets are made with maltitol (see below), which is especially bad for anyone trying to reverse diabetes or struggling with insulin resistance.

Maltitol

Maltitol is a sugar alcohol that, unlike xylitol and erythritol, is cheap and inferior, which is why companies use it to make sugar-free treats. What makes the 'sugar-free' claim misleading on products containing maltitol is that maltitol has quite a high glycaemic index (GI). The glycaemic index measures how a carbohydrate-containing food raises blood sugar levels. To put maltitol into perspective, table sugar has a GI of 60, maltitol syrup has a GI of 56 and maltitol powder a GI of 36.

Soy lecithin/protein

Soy, being one of the most genetically modified crops on earth, has no place in any healthy diet. Soy lecithin is one of the most ubiquitous additives, and is used primarily as an emulsifier. It contains pesticides and solvents, so if you are conscientious about decreasing your exposure to toxins, you should definitely give it a miss.[*]

Vegetable oils

Vegetable seed oils are high in omega-6 fats and contribute to inflammation. Avoid them.

Artificial colouring

In 2010, in a 58-page report titled 'Food dyes: A rainbow of risks', the Center for Science in the Public Interest revealed that nine of the food dyes currently approved for use in the United States are linked to health issues ranging from cancer and hyperactivity to allergy-like reactions – and these results were from studies conducted by the chemical industry itself.[†] Any foods containing artificial colourants should be given a wide berth, whether you're Banting or not.

Processed foods

Most of the foods you consume in a day are processed in one way or another.

- There are two types of processing: mechanical and chemical.
- Mechanical processing includes, for example, making butter from milk or grinding beef to make mince. These processes involve a single food, a real food that still contains only one

---

[*] 'Soy alert!', Weston A. Price Foundation, available at http://www.westonaprice.org/soy-alert/ (last accessed September 2015).

[†] Sarah Kobylewski and Michael F. Jacobson, 'Food dyes: A rainbow of risks', Center for Science in the Public Interest, June 2010, available at http://cspinet.org/new/pdf/food-dyes -rainbow-of-risks.pdf (last accessed September 2015).

ingredient and has had nothing added to it. It is still in its natural form, has its natural taste and is good to eat.

- Chemical processing is generally what we are referring to when we tell you to avoid processed foods. These foods are made from refined ingredients and contain artificial additives.
- Highly processed foods contain preservatives to give them a longer shelf life or to prevent rotting, colourants to give them a specific colour, flavourants to give them an artificial taste, and even texturants.
- Processed foods are the convenient, ready packaged, boxed, highly refined and usually cheaper foods.
- They include: baked goodies, such as bagels, burger and hot-dog buns, all types of bread, croissants, doughnuts, cakes, tarts, cookies and muffins; deli items like pies, pastries, sausage rolls and cold meats; processed meats and cheeses like viennas and individually wrapped cheeses; sauces like cook-in sauces, packet soups and stock cubes; canned foods, such as corned beef, sweet-corn and baked beans; bottled items, such as vegetable and canola oils, tomato sauce, mustard, chutney, mayonnaise, salad dressings and marinades; and foods in tubs, such as margarine, liver pastes, dips, low-fat cream cheese and low-fat yoghurt.

Why is eating processed food bad?

- Processed food is made to be addictive.
- It blocks your body's ability to burn fat and triggers food cravings.
- It hijacks your brain biochemistry, causing an intense dopamine release that leads to addiction to that food.
- Processed foods are usually loaded with sugar and high-fructose corn syrup. Studies have shown that sugar has devastating effects on our metabolism,[*] can lead to insulin resistance, increase tri-

---

[*] Kimber L. Stanhope, Jean-Marc Schwarz, and Peter J. Havel, 'Adverse metabolic effects of dietary fructose: Results from recent epidemiological, clinical, and mechanistic studies', *Current Opinion in Lipidology*, 24(3), June 2013: 198–206, available at http://www.ncbi. nlm.nih.gov/pmc/articles/PMC4251462/ (last accessed September 2015).

glyceride levels, increase levels of harmful cholesterol and lead to fat accumulation in the liver and abdominal cavity.[*]
- Processed foods also have a negative effect on our gut microbiome, which plays an essential role in our overall health.

BANTING ON A BUDGET

Many people are put off by the perceived expense of this lifestyle. They see all the fancy Banting products, from special flours to special sweeteners, and they wonder how they are going to afford it all. But what a lot of newcomers don't realise is that Banting is not about baking fancy and costly low-carb breads, cakes and treats.

This lifestyle is about eating fresh, real food. If done properly, Banting can actually save you money. So, in this section we'll give you some pointers to help make Banting fit your budget.

Basic grocery list

Make a shopping list and keep to simple, straightforward and fresh foods like:

Eggs	Any kind
Fresh meat (not processed)	Any kind you like to eat: chicken, beef mince, pork, offal, mutton, lamb, etc.
Fresh seafood	From the green list: hake, sole, sardines, tuna in water, pilchards in brine (note that pilchards in tomato sauce are not recommended, as the added sauces contain sugar and unhealthy ingredients), etc.
Fresh or frozen vegetables (in season)	Any kind you like to eat: broccoli, cauliflower, green beans, cabbage, mushrooms, onions, spinach, baby marrow, salad ingredients like cucumber, tomato, lettuce, etc.

---

[*] Kimber L. Stanhope, *et al*, 'Consuming fructose-sweetened, not glucose-sweetened, beverages increases visceral adiposity and lipids and decreases insulin sensitivity in overweight/obese humans', *Journal of Clinical Investigation*, 119(5), May 2009: 1322–1334, available at http://www.ncbi.nlm.nih.gov/pmc/articles/PMC2673878/ (last accessed September 2015).

Fresh fruits in season (if you are carb tolerant)	Strawberries, blackberries, blueberries
Dairy	Full-cream milk, cream, cheese, full-cream yoghurt, pure butter
Extras	Herbs and spices (watch out for those with hidden sugar), extra-virgin olive oil, coconut oil, raw nuts and seeds (green list only)

Shopping tips

- Do not stray from your shopping list. Only buy what you have planned to buy. Take a pen and a calculator along with you to mark off the items you have placed in your trolley and calculate how much you have spent, so that you can stay within your budget.
- Once you have established your budget, draw the exact cash instead of taking your debit or credit card with you. Leaving your bank cards at home will make you even more aware of what you put into the trolley.
- Eat satiating, low-carb foods before you go grocery shopping. If you are hungry, you will end up buying all the wrong foods.
- Make sure that you are well hydrated. Take a bottle of water with you if you must, to avoid buying fizzy or inappropriate drinks because you are thirsty.
- Stick to the aisles on the perimeter of the store, where all the fresh vegetables, fruits and meat are kept. Although watch out for the bakeries and delis that are sometimes located in these areas too!
- Avoid the centre aisles, as this is where most of the processed and packaged foods are kept.
- Give yourself a time frame in which to complete your shopping. Shopping when you're in a hurry or when time is limited will ensure you only buy what you need.
- Shop alone. Children can easily distract you and bully you into buying junk food and other unnecessary items.
- If you have to buy a special flour or ingredient, rather visit the

factory outlet. It will be much cheaper than buying it at a health shop, pharmacy or supermarket.

EATING OUT AND SOCIALISING MADE EASY

We don't expect you to give up eating out and socialising, so here are some handy tips to help you navigate any potential pitfalls.

Tips for eating out at a restaurant
Choose the right restaurant

- Plan ahead and make sure that the restaurant has a variety of dishes from which you can choose.
- Most restaurants these days have their menu online. Download the menu at home and decide in advance what you are going to eat.
- Look out for restaurants that have a salad bar where you can dish up your own salad.
- Many Banting-friendly restaurants and bistros have popped up in the last two years, so familiarise yourself with the available options.
- Avoid so-called 'all you can eat' restaurants; they are setting you up for failure.
- Takeaway places are not restaurants and will not have Banting-friendly foods.

Before you leave the house

- Make a reservation so that you don't end up waiting at the bar for a table and hit the drinks.
- When you make the reservation, ask the manager upfront if they are willing to prepare your meal in pure butter or grill your food.
- Ask for a table as far away from the kitchen as possible to escape the smell of all those not-so-Banting-friendly foods.
- Don't starve yourself the whole day if you know you are going

to eat out. Eat something light at home at least an hour before going out, but make sure that these are satiating foods.
- If possible, take your own salad dressing or Banting mayonnaise from home. Don't expect the restaurant to have any Banting-friendly salad dressings or mayonnaise.

When you sit down at the table
- Remember why you are there: to enjoy a relaxed evening with friends or family, not to be tempted by food.
- Politely send the bread basket away and order a glass of water immediately. Sometimes we mistake thirst for hunger. You can also ask for Banting-bread options.
- If you already know what you are going to order, tell your waiter that you are ready to order and don't even look at the menu. Looking at the menu again may change your mind, and you could end up choosing something else that will have a negative effect on your weight loss and health.

When ordering your meal
- Don't be shy to ask your waiter questions and insist that they cook your meal the way you want it cooked.
- Don't order platters, combos or any meals that may come with extras you don't want.
- Replace chips with salad or vegetables, and leave out the onion rings.
- Don't order vegetables that come in creamy sauces, such as creamed spinach, as the sauces are often made with white flour. In fact, leave off any fancy sauces.
- Ask for your meat to be grilled with salt and pepper, no marinades.
- Ordering a starter first instead of heading straight for the main can have the effect of filling you up, meaning you don't need a main. Alternatively, you could opt for a starter as a main meal.

- Do not order any dessert, and watch your drinks. Keep to red wine or clean spirits like whisky with soda water, and remember moderation is always key.
- If you are out for breakfast, opt for eggs, bacon and fried tomato, no toast.

When your meal arrives

- There is no need to rush your meal; it's not a race.
- No matter the size of the meal, only eat until satisfied.
- Eat slowly, and after each bite put your knife and fork down and finish chewing before you pick them up for the next bite.
- Concentrate on the conversation and not your food. The more you talk between bites, the better. The longer you take to eat, the more time your brain will have to register when you are full.
- When you are finished, if there is still food on your plate, ask your waiter to remove it and get you a doggy bag. Don't let the plate sit in front of you, tempting you to take another bite.

Tips for socialising (dinner parties and braais)

- Ask the host if there is anything you can bring. If it's a braai, offer to make a Banting-friendly salad. At least then you can eat your own meat and salad, and no one will even notice you did not eat anything else.
- Eat something light but satiating about an hour before you go out. This way you ensure that you won't overeat at the dinner party, and you won't be as tempted to munch on the pre-dinner snacks. Good examples are fat/protein combinations such as cheese, sardines, pilchards, mackerel, droëwors, etc.
- If there are no Banting options, make clever choices when dishing your meal. Have more salad and a little bit of whatever else there is. The salad will make your plate look deceptively fuller. Or opt for more vegetables over bread, for example.
- Avoid having dessert.

- You can't tell your hosts how to cook or prepare their meals. Next time, invite them around to your house and introduce them to your lifestyle. You might just convert them.
- This is not meant to be a restrictive diet. It's a lifestyle change. It all comes down to making the right choices. The most important thing to remember is to have fun and enjoy the precious moments with friends and family.

PART 4

FREQUENTLY
ASKED QUESTIONS

I'm gluten intolerant or I have coeliac disease, can I Bant?

Gluten is the protein composite found in wheat and related grains. The best part about the LCHF/Banting lifestyle is that we remove wheat and related grains from our diet completely, so someone who is sensitive to gluten or who has coeliac disease can Bant with ease. In fact, this should be the eating plan they need to follow.

I'm on medication for cholesterol/diabetes/depression/ blood pressure/etc. Since I started Banting I feel much better, can I stop taking it now?

If you are on any prescribed medication at all, only reduce your meds or stop them with your doctor's help. It is not safe to just stop taking prescribed medication, as this could have negative health effects. However, it is important to reduce or stop medications if they begin to produce side-effects. For example, persons with diabetes (either type 1 or type 2) will need less insulin on this eating plan. And the same applies to blood-pressure medications in many.

Will an LCHF diet help with type 2 diabetes?

As type 2 diabetes is a disease of too much insulin, treatment should involve reducing insulin production in the body. It would, therefore, make sense to restrict or remove from our diet foods that have the greatest effect on increasing blood insulin concentrations, namely carbohydrates.

Numerous studies have shown that refined carbohydrate consumption is associated with health problems, specifically the metabolic syndrome. Numerous studies have shown that low-carb diets are more effective than low-fat diets in achieving weight loss, as well as greater improvement in other health markers, including cholesterol concentrations, blood pressure and blood sugar.[*]

Lowering our intake of obvious sugars is clearly beneficial in controlling blood glucose. We recommend that diabetics undertake a low-carb diet with the assistance of a supportive health-care practitioner.

I have high cholesterol, can I Bant?

Fear of 'cholesterol' is the planned direct consequence of the pharmaceutical industry's desire to encourage the use of cholesterol-lowering drugs ('statins') by as many people as possible.

But it is not 'cholesterol' that damages our arteries, causing us to have heart attacks and strokes. It is the eating of high-carbohydrate diets by those with insulin resistance/diabetes/metabolic syndrome that causes the blood abnormalities that damage our arteries. (See Introduction.)

---

[*] See, for example: Bonnie J. Brehm, *et al*, 'A randomized trial comparing a very low carbohydrate diet and a calorie-restricted low fat diet on body weight and cardiovascular risk factors in healthy women', *Journal of Clinical Endocrinology & Metabolism*, 88(4), April 2003: 1617–23; Y. Wady Aude, *et al*, 'The national cholesterol education program diet vs a diet lower in carbohydrates and higher in protein and monounsaturated fat: A randomized trial', *Archives of Internal Medicine*, 164(19), October 2004: 2141–6; W.S. Yancy Jr, *et al*, 'A low-carbohydrate, ketogenic diet versus a low-fat diet to treat obesity and hyperlipidemia: A randomized, controlled trial', *Annals of Internal Medicine*, 140(10), May 2004: 769–77.

So the question is not whether or not you have 'high cholesterol'. It is whether or not you are insulin resistant. Table 1 on p. 11 lists the blood tests that can help you decide whether or not you are insulin resistant. If you are insulin resistant, the key to your future health is to eat the Banting diet described in this book.

What about non-alcoholic fatty liver disease (NAFLD)?

NAFLD is caused by drinking fructose-loaded soft drinks and eating excessive quantities of refined carbohydrates. Many jump to the conclusion that fat causes fatty liver disease, but this is not true. Studies have shown that liver fat can be significantly reduced in a very short space of time by eating a low-carb diet.[*]

I don't have a gallbladder. What about all that fat?

As we have already seen, 'all that fat' is not as much fat as you think. The reason people worry about eating fat after having their gallbladder removed is because they don't realise that the liver actually produces the bile which assists in the digestion and absorption of fats. Bile flows out of the liver through a duct that joins with another duct coming from the gallbladder. Between meals, bile salts are stored in the gallbladder, and only a small amount of bile flows into the intestine.

When we remove the gallbladder, we remove the reservoir, but bile is still being produced by the liver. Instead of being stored, the bile is simply delivered directly into the small intestine.

Will I get gallstones if I Bant?

Research indicates that it's not the consumption of too much fat that causes gallstones, but *too little* fat. Contrary to what we've been

---

[*] H. Bian, *et al*, 'Effects of dietary interventions on liver volume in humans', *Obesity*, 22(4), April 2014: 989–995; Browning, *et al*, 'Short-term weight loss and hepatic triglyceride reduction'; Rebecca C. Schugar and Peter A. Crawford, 'Low-carbohydrate ketogenic diets, glucose homeostasis, and nonalcoholic fatty liver disease', *Current Opinion in Clinical Nutrition & Metabolic Care*, 15(4), July 2012: 374–80.

told, it's a diet high in grains, sugar and starch that leads to gall-bladder problems.

The purpose of the gallbladder is to store bile that it receives from the liver. Bile emulsifies fat. When there is too little fat in the diet, the gallbladder does not contract to release bile and therefore does not empty properly. Bile acids are made from cholesterol. When the gallbladder does not empty, the bile in it stagnates and thickens and its cholesterol concentration increases, resulting in the formation of cholesterol crystals and eventually gallstones.

You need fat in your diet for the gallbladder to function properly. If you have existing gallstones, eating fat may cause a problem initially, and it may be necessary to remove the stones and the gallbladder. But Banting is not the cause of the problem, and it is likely that at some point existing gallstones would have become a problem even on a low-fat diet and would have required medical intervention.

When I have PMS I crave everything sweet, why is this?

During PMS the stress hormone cortisol spikes and the feel-good hormone serotonin dips. This fluctuation can lead to craving the wrong foods, especially sugar, because sugar boosts serotonin levels in the brain. The best way to combat this is to eliminate these foods from your diet so that your hormone and blood sugar levels can stabilise.

I'm pregnant/breastfeeding, can I Bant?

Remember that each time you eat carbohydrates, your blood glucose rises and this exposes the foetus to a high blood glucose concentration. But insulin from the mother does not cross the placenta to the foetus. So your unborn baby must make its own insulin to lower the elevated blood glucose that your eating caused. Repeated exposure to high blood glucose levels causes the foetus to become increasingly insulin resistant, fatter, and at increased risk of future obesity and type 2 diabetes. At birth, insulin resistant babies are at risk of developing sudden falls in blood glucose concentrations – neonatal hypoglycaemia. A dangerous condition that has become all too common in mother overeating carbohydrates during pregnancy.

Cutting out unhealthy refined carbohydrates, processed foods and sugar is definitely advisable for breastfeeding moms to benefit both you and your baby. So, although you may not want to embark on a fully ketogenic (LCHF) diet at this time, following a low-carb, healthy-fat diet is recommended.

What is keto flu?

Otherwise known as carb flu, keto flu is basically carbohydrate withdrawal. Symptoms can include dull headaches, fatigue, dizziness, moodiness and aching joints. Some people describe feeling as if they are in a mental 'fog'.

Some people feel a little under the weather for only a day or two, but others may take a few weeks to adapt. Some become convinced during this phase that they are unable to function without significant carbohydrates and throw in the towel. If you know what to expect, you can minimise the effects and push through.

Will I become constipated if I Bant?

Only some people who have not experienced constipation before become constipated when they start Banting.

For beginner Banters, constipation is usually a transient problem that resolves within a couple of weeks, if not sooner. One way to combat this is to drink enough water.

Taking a course of good-quality probiotics can really help. Probiotics are bacteria that can be bought in supplement form. Different probiotics work for different health conditions, so ask your pharmacist or health shop which will be best for you.

Be sure that you are eating sufficient vegetable matter as well as sufficient fat. Many people start out on a diet by being too restrictive or by eliminating a large amount of vegetable matter and therefore fibre. Some people find that supplementing with psyllium husk helps to relieve constipation. Others find coconut oil to be especially helpful. Regular exercise may also help with bowel motility, even a brisk 15-minute walk.

Keep in mind that most commonly used laxatives are gut irritants and will damage the lining of the gut. Remember that we are trying to heal the gut, not damage it further. If your attempts to get your bowels working do not yield results, see your doctor, but preferably one who understands the low-carb lifestyle.

I've been extremely nauseous since I began Banting, what can I do to reduce this symptom?

Nausea may initially be a symptom of keto flu. If you are continuously nauseous on Banting, you may be consuming too much fat. Check your fat intake and don't add extra fat to already fatty foods. Drinking ginger tea may help to alleviate nausea, as ginger is a natural anti-emetic.

My mouth tastes and smells funny, why is this? What can I do to reduce these symptoms?

One of the results of cutting carbs is that our bodies start to use fat for energy. This results in ketones being excreted in the breath and urine. The good news is that this does not last indefinitely and usually subsides after a couple of weeks. In the meanwhile, be sure to drink enough water, brush your teeth regularly to freshen up your mouth, and use natural breath fresheners like mint, parsley, cloves, cinnamon and ginger.

I've had serious headaches since I started Banting, why and what can I do about it?

When new to a low-carb diet, a headache may manifest for a number of reasons. The most common cause is a loss of sodium, and this may be quickly rectified by mixing a quarter teaspoon of natural salt in a glass of water and drinking it. Another cause of headaches is dehydration, so make sure you are drinking enough good-quality water.

Always try to resolve a headache naturally with a bit of rest and a head and neck massage before reaching for medication. Remember, we are trying to clean up our bodies, not add any more chemicals to the mix.

I've been experiencing leg cramps since I started Banting, why and what can I do?

Dietary deficiency is the most common cause of this problem and can be remedied by upping mineral and electrolyte intake.

Be aware that not all aches and pains and abnormalities can be attributed to beginning a low-carb diet. Sitting or standing in one position for too long can cause muscle cramps. Arthritis, varicose veins, fibromyalgia and hormone imbalances can contribute to leg cramps too. It is important to check with your health-care practitioner if you experience any persistent problems.

I've felt bloated since I started Banting, why and what can I do about it?

It is unusual to experience bloating once you have eliminated grains and refined carbs, but some people may be sensitive to FODMAPs (fermentable oligosaccharides, disaccharides, monosaccharides and polyols), a collection of foods to which a surprisingly large number of people are sensitive, especially after years of mistreating the gut. These include vegetables such as onions, garlic, cabbage, broccoli, etc. If you are experiencing bloating, you may want to cut out these vegetables for a while. Dairy can be a culprit too, and we would recommend cutting back on this first. A good probiotic could also be very helpful.

I seem to be losing a lot of hair, is my diet responsible?

The root of the hair is supplied nutrients by the follicle, which is a small pocket below the surface of the skin. Hair has two growth phases: the anagen phase, in which hair can grow steadily for two to three years, and the telogen phase, which is a resting phase in which the hair stops growing for up to three months. Approximately 10 per cent of hair goes into the resting phase, while the other 90 per cent keeps growing. At the end of the rest stage, new hair starts growing and pushes the old hair out. If a person consumes less energy than the body needs, or removes crucial nutrients, this creates stress in the body and more hair follicles than normal go into the resting phase. This is possibly because the body does not have sufficient energy or nutrients to support the growth phase. Once the stress has passed, hair growth starts again. If a large percentage of hair was in the telogen phase, the new growth will result in greater hair loss.

How can I avoid sugar cravings?

A craving is the brain's need for reward. It does not mean your body needs sugar. Craving is not the same as hunger, but a craving on top of hunger will feel a whole lot worse and you will more easily give in to temptation. So, make sure you are eating enough at mealtimes to feel satiated. **Remember, sugar is a drug, not a food.** Treat your sugar cravings as drug withdrawal. Sugar addiction is the toughest addiction of all. You have to treat it by practising complete abstinence from sugar.

Can I drink diet soda?

No. Diet sodas are loaded with all sorts of chemicals and unhealthy artificial sweeteners. Diet drinks have no nutritional value.

Can I drink alcohol?

Alcohol is a toxin that can't be used by the body and that needs to be processed by the liver. While it's being processed, fat burning is put on hold. Alcohol should only be consumed occasionally. Refer to the yellow list in Part 8 for allowed alcohol.

Can I have fruit juice and dried fruit?

There is evidence that when fructose found in commercial fruit juices as added sugar is consumed in excess amounts, it can lead to health problems such as obesity, type 2 diabetes, metabolic syndrome and Non-Alcoholic Fatty Liver Disease (NAFLD). Store-bought fruit juices are processed – they contain all sorts of other ingredients that are unhealthy. If you make a fresh homemade fruit juice, the amount of fruit you will have to use to make up one glass will contain too much sugar. Most dried fruit is also loaded with sugar and other harmful ingredients. We therefore don't advocate having fruit juice or dried fruit at all.

Can I eat soy products?

Genetically engineered soy is highly processed and very harmful to your health. Soy isoflavones are phyto-endocrine disruptors, which means that at dietary levels they can prevent ovulation and stimulate the growth of cancer cells. Eating as little as 30 grams (about four tablespoons) of soy per day can result in hypothyroidism with symptoms of lethargy, constipation, weight gain and fatigue. The bottom line is that soy is found in almost all processed and junk foods, so if you avoid these foods, you can successfully avoid soy.

Can I use whey protein?

If you are eating correctly there should be no reason you require additional protein. Protein powders are highly processed, usually contain artificial flavourings and sweeteners and are often heated to the point that the protein is denatured, which makes it nearly impossible for the body to recognise and use it. Rather eat whole protein foods like liver, sardines and eggs.

How much fruit can I eat?

Unfortunately fruit is on the orange list, so if you are trying to lose weight, reduce your insulin levels or have a metabolic disorder, it is better to give fruit a miss. An occasional treat is acceptable, but try to stick to the lower-carb options like berries, and remember it is all part of your daily carb count.

How much coffee with cream can I drink?

The best answer here would be none. Cream is energy dense and, if you are trying to lose weight, too much of it may stall your weight loss. You need to experiment with yourself, but if you are eating correctly and not losing weight, the cream needs to go.

Is drinking iced water bad for you?

It is alleged that iced water will solidify the fat that you eat, which will slow down digestion, line the intestines and cause cancer. This is simply untrue. Your body is an ace self-regulator, regulating its core temperature between 36.5 and 37 degrees. From the moment the water enters your mouth, heat transfer from your body begins to warm it up, and within a few minutes the temperature of the iced water equals that of your body.

Is it safe to use frozen fruit and vegetables?

Some people argue that frozen vegetables are processed because they go through a mechanical process, but some frozen vegetables are actually more nutrient dense than the fresh produce available to us. In many cases the 'fresh' fruit and vegetables on the shop shelf have been harvested long before they are actually ripe, which means they were not able to reach their peak nutritional potential.

Once picked, fruit and vegetables begin to lose nutritional content. By the time the produce reaches the shelves – after being transported long distances, often irradiated, and kept in cold storage – it has lost quite a bit of its nutritional content.

For freezing, fruit and vegetables are picked when they are at their maximum ripeness and are then frozen immediately, in most cases on the same day. The quick freezing process does affect some of the vitamin content, but it locks or freezes most of the nutrients in place.

Can I snack between meals, and which snacks are Banting friendly?

Rather don't snack between meals. The need to snack is a myth perpetuated by the food industry to make you eat more. If you are trying to lose weight, then you need to give your body time to lower insulin and start releasing fat. Even so-called 'Banting-friendly' snacks will make you release insulin.

What are BPCs and 'fat bombs', and can you lose weight on them?

A BPC or bulletproof coffee is a cup of filter coffee with a tablespoon of coconut oil and a tablespoon of butter whisked into it to create a foamy hot drink. They serve a purpose for athletes requiring additional energy, but for people trying to lose weight and learn better eating habits they are best left alone. 'Fat bombs' are just an excuse to eat sweets. There are a number of recipes, but all result in some form of fat-dense bonbon.

I'm vegetarian, can I Bant?

Yes, many vegetarians successfully eat an LCHF diet, especially if they eat dairy products and eggs. It may be a little challenging at times to get enough protein, but it can be done. Refer to Part 7 for a meal plan.

Why can I not use artificial sweeteners?

Artificial sweeteners get a lot of bad press for many valid reasons. They can impair the innate ability to regulate caloric intake; simply put, they can make you eat more. The best thing you can do for yourself is to cut out all sweet stuff.

What are 'units', I see people say you need to 'get your units'?

Some groups have created meal plans comprising food units, for example 6F/3P/2C, where 'F' stands for fats, 'P' for protein and 'C' for carbs. The unit system divides food up into single macronutrients, but often our food cannot be divided into single macronutrients. Most of the foods we consume contain at least two of the three macronutrients. If you do need to fine-tune your diet and track your food, then counting the actual macronutrients in the foods you eat is the safest and most effective way of doing it.

Do I have to eat breakfast?

Breakfast is great for some and not so great for others. Insisting that someone eat breakfast to achieve weight loss could be the very thing that makes it harder for him or her to lose weight. Some people feel and do better not eating breakfast, and there is no reason for them to change.

Can I have a cheat day?

Banting is a lifestyle. The purpose is not just weight loss; people who undertake to eat this way are encouraged to embrace it as a long-term lifestyle change. It therefore makes no sense to revert to bad habits once a week. Many people who cut out sugar and carbohydrates do so because they are addicted to them. You wouldn't tell a recovering alcoholic that it's okay to have a drink once a week, or an ex-smoker one cigarette a week. It simply does not make sense to cheat. Consistency is the key here.

What is the blood-type diet?

The blood-type diet is based on the misguided belief that the optimal diet for any individual depends on that individual's blood type. There is NO reasonable scientific basis for the claims that diet should be based on blood type. In 2013, researchers examined the data from over a thousand studies and yet did not find one well-designed study to support the blood-type theory.[*]

What about the alkaline diet?

Proponents of this diet claim that replacing acid-forming foods with alkaline foods can improve health and fight serious diseases like cancer. While the alkaline diet is quite healthy, the claims about the mechanism behind the diet are simply not supported by science.

If I skip a meal will my body enter starvation mode?

People who do not eat, lose weight. Their metabolisms do not shut down. From an evolutionary perspective, it would be extremely disadvantageous for the survival of the human species if after one or two skipped meals our metabolisms shut down, leaving us lethargic and unable to hunt for our next meal. Another aspect of this myth is that if we skip meals our bodies will scavenge our muscles for energy. This is nonsense. Human beings store fat for good reason. When we do not have a supply of food, our bodies' preferred source of fuel is fat, not muscle.

---

[*] L. Cusack, *et al*, 'Blood type diets lack supporting evidence: a systematic review', *American Journal of Clinical Nutrition*, May 2013, doi: 10.3945/?ajcn.113.058693

PART 5

TROUBLESHOOTING STALLING OR WEIGHT GAIN

In this section we'll take a look at why either your weight loss is stalling or you are gaining weight on Banting, and what you can do about it.

A weight-loss stall is when you do not lose any body fat for more than two consecutive weeks. Sometimes you just need to tweak and adjust a little bit to speed things up again. Remember that you didn't gain all that weight in two weeks. It took you a long time to gain it and it may take you a long time to lose it. Any loss is greater than no loss, as long as it's consistent.

Remember, you don't have to walk this road alone. We have a support system in place to help you recognise and correct pitfalls; all it takes is a consultation with us either online or face to face. Whenever you feel that you cannot deal with the issues on your own, you know where to find help (see page 171).

Scenario 1: Eating the wrong foods

Are you eating only from the green list? Or have a few orange- or red-list food items sneaked into your meals? Even though orange foods are quality foods, they are high in carbohydrates.

Solution: If you keep to the green list all of the time, you can rest assured that you are eating quality, real food. Try to commit to live at least 90 per cent off the green list. Remember that once you are close to goal weight, or you have reached your goal weight, you can start introducing some orange-list foods into your diet, but only if you do not start gaining weight again.

Scenario 2: Eating too much from the green list

A few people complain that they have stalled or gained weight despite strictly adhering to only green-list foods. There are two possible explanations for this. Either they are profoundly insulin resistant without realising it (Solution 1), or they are simply eating way more food than their body really needs (Solution 2).

Solution 1: If you are profoundly insulin resistant or suspect that you might be, consider eating more of the foods with the *LIND* (low insulinogenic, nutrient dense) sign next to them on the green list. These have a lower insulinogenic effect on the body. You can also try out Meal Plan 1 (see Part 7) for profound insulin resistance and nutritional ketosis to help you get started.

Solution 2: Remember that too much of a good thing is not such a good thing. Eating too much food will result in a stall or in weight gain. Check how much fat, protein and carbohydrate you should eat per day to lose weight. First try Tool 1 (see section on meal planning), but if you are still not losing weight, you might want to consider getting your macro requirements professionally calculated at one of our clinics (Tool 2). Once you have established how much you should be eating per day, you can track your food intake. This will ensure that you do not overeat.

Scenario 3: Eating too much dairy

Some women in particular find that they start to gain weight when they consume dairy products like cheese, cream and milk. Some dairy products, irrespective of whether they are lower in carbohydrate or higher in protein, can increase insulin levels, resulting in fat storage.

Solution: Before you go mad and start cutting out all dairy from your diet, first look at the green list and choose only those items with the *LIND* sign next to them. These dairy foods will have a low insulinogenic effect. If you have tried and tested and tweaked and you still don't have the results you were hoping for, then you can cut out dairy completely. You might just be sensitive to lactose, the natural sugar found in dairy.

Scenario 4: Thinking 'LCHF equals unlimited fats'

Some people equate high fat with unlimited fat, adding fat to fat, for example having three eggs (which already contain fat), half an avocado and a bullet coffee for breakfast. This is fine if it satiates so much that you do not need to eat again until dinner time. But if eating so much fat does not satiate you, then it may cause you to eat too many calories and so, inevitably, gain weight.

Solution: LCHF does not mean you can eat unlimited fat; it means your fat ratio should be the highest. If you are obese and you have plenty of stored body fat, then you obviously want to burn the stored fat and not the fat you consume. Remember that your fat intake should be just enough to satisfy you – to take away your hunger and so to allow you to eat fewer calories.

Scenario 5: Falling for Banting-friendly and sugar-free products

Banting-friendly, low-carb and sugar-free foods are where hidden sugars and harmful ingredients lurk. By reaching for these products, without realising it, Banters end up replacing one old bad eating habit with an even worse one.

Solution: Eat *real food*. No quick-fix product, no matter how attractive it looks, will benefit your health and waistline like real food does. Once again, if you keep to the green list and only eat real fresh food, you can be assured you are eating nutritious food. If you don't buy the fake products, you won't eat them.

Scenario 6: Always snacking

For many years dietitians and nutritionists urged us to rather eat six meals a day. Some advocated three larger meals with three snacks in between, while others argued for six small meals throughout the day. Continuous snacking or grazing leads to weight gain, as it keeps us in a perpetually hyperinsulinaemic state.

Solution: Some Banters eat only three meals a day, while others eat only two, and they *still lose weight*. Snacking is not encouraged. Even though you may be snacking on healthy foods, they gobble up your daily macronutrient allowance and before you can say 'fat', you've gained weight. If you are a snacker, keep a food diary for a week or log and track your intake, so that you can see how easy it is to reach your limits if you include simple snacks. If you're snacking because you're hungry, then you clearly did not eat enough at your last meal or you ate the wrong foods (which caused you to get hungry sooner, like high carbs).

Scenario 7: Fasting

One of the most effective ways to overcome a weight-loss stall and decrease hunger and cravings is to practise intermittent fasting. Intermittent fasting is a pattern of eating and then making a conscious decision to skip certain meals. Before body fat can be efficiently burned, glycogen stores must be used up. Although lowering carbohydrate intake is helpful, it takes about 10 to 12 hours to use up glycogen stores, so if you are eating three meals a day, you may not be tapping into your glycogen stores enough. Abstaining from food for 10 to 12 hours will give your body time to use up the glycogen stores and start using stored fat for energy.

There are several different intermittent fasting methods. Most people already fast every day, while they are sleeping. Intermittent fasting can be as simple as extending that fast a little longer. You can do this by skipping breakfast and eating your first meal at noon. You would then be fasting for 16 hours. This can be extended to skip lunch, too, making it a 24-hour fast. Some people fast for an entire day or longer. Intermittent fasting can be adapted to the individual. Longer fasts are generally more beneficial for very insulin-resistant people, while shorter fasts are more suitable for those who do not have a lot of weight to lose.

No food is consumed during fasting, but it is important to stay well hydrated. Black tea, coffee, water and bone broth are all acceptable fluids to drink during a fast.

Scenario 8: Cheating

Cheat days, where you eat whatever you feel like one day a week or once every second week, are a sure way to set yourself back. If you are in nutritional ketosis, chances are you will fall out of ketosis and set yourself back at least three days. While you probably won't gain weight after one 'small' cheat every second month or so, frequent cheating with foods like pizza and cake that are high in carbs and bad fats can lead to weight gain.

Solution: First and foremost, don't cheat! Think about it this way: Is it really worth feeling terrible the next day or falling out of ketosis? What could possibly be better tasting and more satisfying than real, fresh food that you've cooked yourself? Those who cheat often and cannot resist junk food or sweets are most likely food addicts, and that's serious. We suggest you seek professional help if this applies to you.

Scenario 9: Doing low-carb and low-fat at the same time

Many women, in particular, attempt to do low-carb and low-fat at the same time. This is understandable when you think that we've been told for such a long time that fat is the enemy. We think we can 'play it safe' by doing low-carb with low-fat. While you will lose weight for a short time, it's unsustainable. You will be hungry all the time, which leaves you vulnerable to binge eating. And as soon as you give in to that, you will gain weight.

Solution: Let's be realistic. We know that for some new Banters, especially women, the whole 'fat is good' idea can be a bit overwhelming, and we understand that some people are just not cut out for fatty foods. Remember, you have more than enough fat stored in your body to burn, so ideally starting out with smaller amounts of fat is good.

Scenario 10: Lacking accountability

If you are one of those people who struggle to be consistent, you might want to consider getting a support system to which you can be accountable. If you have to report to someone on a weekly basis, where you get weighed, for example, or meet up for a group session, you are more likely to keep to your healthy weight-loss routine.

Solution: Sign up to one of our Banting slimming clinics. Not only will you be measured during the course, but the clinic consultant will also keep a watchful eye on you and support you through your weight-loss journey. You can refer to our website for more details (see page 171).

Scenario 11: Too many diets in the past

Have you been a yo-yo dieter in the past 10, 20, 40 years? Have you tried out many different diets, for long or short periods at a time, losing weight and then gaining it all back again? In all likelihood your metabolism is pretty messed up as a result. To expect that the LCHF/Banting lifestyle will fix everything overnight is wishful thinking. Weight loss does not happen overnight in everyone.

Solution: You need to realise that this is a lifestyle change and not one of those quick-fix diets you've tried before. You have to have patience and discipline. Expect to wait for proper results, as these things take time. Your metabolism is messed up and needs to be fixed, which also takes time. Focus more on how you feel and that you are getting healthier.

Scenario 12: Too much stress

While we typically think of stress as a psychological challenge, there are a number of physiological challenges that cause stress, such as insomnia, inflammation, autoimmune disease, too much exercise and dieting. Our bodies respond to all stress in the same way, whether it's physical or psychological.

As long as stress continues, the body is pumping out cortisol, which in turn is telling the body to replenish energy, even if you haven't used any. Cortisol also reduces the ability to burn fat and makes us hungry. Added to this, the foods we crave when stressed are usually high in carbohydrates, the fuel our muscles use during the fight or flight response. Not only does this lead to weight gain, but cortisol also has the ability to mobilise fat from healthier areas and deposit it around the abdomen – contributing to that increasing belly fat.

Solution: Low-strain, moderate exercise is the best stress buster. Moving those muscles fools your body into thinking you are escaping the source of your stress. Even a simple activity like walking or swimming produces a cascade of effects that counter the negative effects of stress hormones, as well as help lower insulin and blood sugar levels.

Devote time to relaxation. Find activities that make you feel relaxed and calm. For some, this could be taking up a hobby or practising meditation or deep-breathing techniques. Taking some time off to read a good book or listen to music will help counter the effects of stress.

Scenario 13: Not enough sleep

There is mounting evidence that people who sleep too little have a higher risk of weight gain and obesity than people who get seven to eight hours of sleep a night. We are talking about people who are regularly getting too little sleep or poor-quality sleep. Insufficient sleep increases appetite because of the effects it has on hunger hormones and metabolism.

Solution: Make a point of going to bed at the same time each night and waking at the same time each morning. Being consistent reinforces the body's sleep–wake cycle and helps promote better sleep at night.

Develop a relaxing ritual before bedtime. Avoid bright lights, TV screens, computers and other technology an hour before bedtime, as well as any activity that causes excitement, stress or anxiety. A relaxing activity may include taking a warm bath or shower, reading a book or listening to soothing music – preferably with the lights dimmed.

Create a room that's ideal for sleeping. Your bedroom should be cool, dark and quiet. Consider using block-out curtains, earplugs, a fan or other devices that create white noise to create an environment that suits your needs. Your mattress and pillow can contribute to better sleep, too. Bedding is subjective, so choose what is most comfortable for you.

Regular physical activity can promote better sleep, helping you to fall asleep faster and to enjoy deeper sleep. Timing is important, though. If you exercise too close to bedtime, you might be too energised to fall asleep.

PART 6

BANTING RECIPES

Please note: The nutritional values given for each recipe are based on the raw ingredients and may differ once the recipe is prepared and cooked.

Conversion chart	
Imperial	*Metric*
¼ tsp	1 ml
½ tsp	2.5 ml
1 tsp	5 ml
1 Tbsp	15 ml
¼ cup	60 ml
½ cup	125 ml
¾ cup	180 ml
1 cup	250 ml

BREAKFAST

Ratatouille with eggs

> Lacto-ovo-vegetarian friendly

Serves 6

4 tsp olive oil
2 medium onions, chopped
1 medium green pepper, deseeded and chopped

4 medium baby marrows, chopped

3 ripe tomatoes, chopped

1 cup chopped aubergine

2 tsp dried mixed herbs

1 tsp xylitol

1 Tbsp Worcestershire sauce

lemon juice and freshly ground black pepper to taste

3 Tbsp chopped fresh parsley

6 eggs

6 slices toasted Banting bread (see recipe on page 128) to serve

1. Heat half the oil in a large frying pan and fry the onions and green pepper for a few minutes until soft.
2. Add the baby marrows, tomatoes and aubergine along with the dried herbs, xylitol and Worcestershire sauce.
3. Fry for a few minutes, then reduce the heat and simmer uncovered for 15–20 minutes.
4. Season with lemon juice and black pepper, and add half the parsley.
5. Make six hollows in the sauce and pour in the rest of the oil.
6. Crack an egg into each hollow. Simmer with the lid on for 4–5 minutes or until the eggs are cooked to your preference. Sprinkle over the rest of the parsley.
7. Spoon an egg and some of the sauce onto each slice of toasted Banting bread.

Nutritional values per	Fat	Protein	Net Carbs
1 serving	26 g	19 g	17 g

Herbed eggs and tomato on toast

Lacto-ovo-vegetarian friendly

Serves 2

2 eggs
2 egg whites
½ cup deseeded and chopped green pepper
1 tsp crushed garlic
½ tsp dried mixed herbs
4 tsp Banting cheeky chutney (see recipe on page 131)
4 cherry tomatoes, halved
2 slices toasted Banting bread (see recipe on page 128)
30 g Cheddar cheese, grated
salt and freshly ground black pepper to taste

1. Break each whole egg into a separate microwaveable bowl and break up the yolks. Add an extra egg white to each and stir lightly.
2. Divide the green pepper, garlic and dried herbs between the bowls and microwave each on high for 60–90 seconds, depending on the power of your microwave.
3. Stir lightly and top each with chutney and tomatoes.
4. Microwave for another 40 seconds on high.
5. Invert the contents of each bowl onto a slice of Banting toast on a microwaveable plate and top with grated cheese (the cooked tomato will now be on the toast with the egg on top of it).
6. Microwave each plate on high for 10–15 seconds to melt the cheese.
7. Season with salt and pepper before serving as breakfast for two.

Nutritional values per	Fat	Protein	Net Carbs
1 serving	27 g	25 g	15 g

Bacon and feta quiche

Serves 4

3 Tbsp butter
1 medium onion, chopped
125 g shoulder bacon, finely chopped
1 cup grated baby marrow
1 tsp crushed garlic
2 cups shredded fresh spinach
½ cup coconut flour
1 tsp baking powder
1 tsp salt
½ tsp freshly ground black pepper
½ tsp paprika
½ tsp ground nutmeg
3 extra-large eggs, whisked
1 cup Greek yoghurt
1 cup crumbled Danish-style feta

1. Preheat the oven to 180 °C and grease a medium quiche or pie dish with butter.
2. Melt the butter in a frying pan and fry the onion, bacon, baby marrow and garlic for 5 minutes.
3. Add the spinach and fry for 1 minute, then remove from the heat and allow to cool.
4. Combine all the remaining ingredients in a large bowl and mix in the spinach mixture.
5. Pour the mixture into the greased dish and bake for 45 minutes.
6. Cut into quarters and serve.

Nutritional values per	Fat	Protein	Net Carbs
1 serving	42 g	27 g	13 g

Quick egg muffins

Flexitarian friendly	

Makes 12 muffins

6 eggs
1 cup sour cream or cream cheese
salt and freshly ground black pepper to taste
1 green pepper, deseeded and chopped
1 red pepper, deseeded and chopped
3 small spring onions, chopped
1 Tbsp coconut oil (or other fat)
1 cup chopped smoked chicken breast
1 cup grated Cheddar cheese
1 cup chopped green-list vegetables (such as spinach, baby marrows, broccoli, mushrooms, etc.)
2 Tbsp chopped fresh herbs (optional)

1. Preheat the oven to 180 °C and grease a muffin tin with butter.
2. Beat the eggs in a large bowl and mix in the sour cream or cream cheese. Season to taste.
3. Sauté the peppers and onions in the coconut oil in a frying pan. Add to the egg mixture.
4. Mix in the remaining ingredients and pour into the muffin tin.
5. Bake for 30 minutes or until golden brown.

Note: These will keep in the fridge for five to six days. They also freeze well.

Nutritional values per	Fat	Protein	Net Carbs
muffin	14 g	6 g	4 g

Chia-seed porridge

Lacto-ovo-vegetarian friendly

Serves 1

25 g dry chia seeds
50 ml coconut cream
1 cup boiling water
1 Tbsp butter
½ tsp vanilla essence
1 Tbsp melted coconut oil
ground cinnamon to taste (optional)

1. In a porridge bowl, mix the chia seeds with the coconut cream and boiling water.
2. Leave the mixture to soak overnight in the fridge.
3. In the morning, warm it up in the microwave and add the butter, vanilla essence and coconut oil.
4. Mix well and sprinkle over some cinnamon if desired.

Nutritional values per	Fat	Protein	Net Carbs
1 serving	52 g	6 g	13 g

Coconut almond porridge

Lacto-ovo-vegetarian friendly

Serves 1

1 large egg
100 ml coconut cream
1 Tbsp desiccated coconut
1 Tbsp almond flour
ground cinnamon to taste
a pinch of salt
1 Tbsp unsalted butter

1. Beat the egg and coconut cream in a mixing bowl, and then add the remaining dry ingredients.
2. Melt the butter in a saucepan, add the egg mixture and stir until thickened to your liking.
3. Serve with a few blueberries and a dash of cream.

Nutritional values per	Fat	Protein	Net Carbs
1 serving (porridge only)	63 g	16 g	11 g

Heba pap

Lacto-ovo-vegetarian friendly

Serves 4

1 cup Heba
3 cups water
a pinch of salt

1. Gently heat the Heba, water and salt in a saucepan on the stove, stirring well.
2. When it begins to boil, remove from the heat and serve.

Nutritional values per	Fat	Protein	Net Carbs
1 serving	14 g	14 g	5 g

Heba porridge

Lacto-ovo-vegetarian friendly

Serves 1

¼ cup Heba
¾ cup boiling water
a pinch of salt

1. Combine the Heba, water and salt in a bowl and stir well.
2. Allow to cool before serving.

Nutritional values per	Fat	Protein	Net Carbs
1 serving	14 g	14 g	5 g

Cream-cheese pancakes

Lacto-ovo-vegetarian friendly

Serves 2

2 extra-large eggs
60 g cream cheese
a pinch of salt
1 Tbsp butter

Topping
2 Tbsp whipped cream
20 blueberries
30 g chopped nuts of your choice

1. In a mixing bowl, beat the eggs and then add the cream cheese and salt, beating until smooth.
2. Melt the butter in a small frying pan. Spoon in the desired amount of mixture depending on the size of pancake you want.
3. Cook over a medium heat until bubbles form on the surface and then flip the pancake to cook the other side.
4. Divide the toppings between the two pancakes and serve.

Nutritional values per	Fat	Protein	Net Carbs
2 pancakes with topping	32 g	12 g	5 g
2 pancakes without topping	27 g	5 g	3 g

Three-minute microwave flax muffin

Makes 1 muffin

3 Tbsp flaxseed flour
a pinch of bicarbonate of soda
a pinch of salt
1 large egg, beaten
1–2 Tbsp water

1. Combine the dry ingredients in a mixing bowl.
2. Add the beaten egg and water, and mix. It should be the consistency of yoghurt. Add more water if needed.
3. Pour the mixture into a coffee mug and microwave on high for 3–4 minutes.
4. Flip out onto a plate and allow to cool.
5. Cut in half, spread with butter and top with some grated cheese to serve.

Note: Create your own flavours. For a chocolate muffin, add 1–2 tsp cocoa powder; for a vanilla flavour, add 1 tsp vanilla essence; for a nutty version, add 1 Tbsp chopped mixed nuts and seeds; and for a coconut muffin, replace 1 Tbsp flaxseed flour with 1 Tbsp milled coconut flour.

Nutritional values per	Fat	Protein	Net Carbs
1 portion	21 g	15 g	3 g

Banting breakfast granola

Lacto-ovo-vegetarian friendly

Makes about 1.1 kg

1 cup chopped almonds
½ cup chopped hazelnuts
½ cup chopped walnuts
½ cup slivered almonds
½ cup flaked coconut
¼ cup chia seeds
½ cup pumpkin seeds
½ cup sunflower seeds
75 ml melted coconut oil
1 tsp ground cinnamon
1 tsp vanilla essence
1 tsp ground ginger
½ tsp ground nutmeg
½ tsp salt

1. Preheat the oven to 120 °C.
2. In a large bowl, combine all the ingredients, mixing very well to make sure everything has a fine coating of oil and spices.
3. Spread the granola on a baking tray and bake for about 30 minutes or until golden throughout.
4. Remove from the oven and allow to cool fully before storing in a clean, airtight container.

Nutritional values per	Fat	Protein	Net Carbs
100 g	67 g	19 g	14 g

LUNCH

Crustless cheese, bacon and vegetable tart

Serves 4

125 g shoulder bacon, finely chopped
1 tsp butter
3 extra-large eggs, whisked
200 g full-fat cottage cheese
1 tsp finely grated Parmesan cheese
1 clove garlic, crushed
a pinch of ground cumin (optional)
salt and freshly ground black pepper to taste
500 g green-list vegetables (such as spinach, baby marrows, broccoli, mushrooms, etc.)
1 small onion, finely chopped
60 g mozzarella cheese, grated
½ tsp paprika

1. Preheat the oven to 180 °C. Lightly grease a medium quiche or pie dish with butter.
2. Lightly fry the bacon in the butter.
3. Mix the eggs, cottage cheese, Parmesan cheese, garlic, cumin, salt and pepper in a bowl and set aside.
4. Peel and finely chop the vegetables, and spread them evenly on the bottom of the greased dish.
5. Sprinkle over the chopped onion.
6. Add the bacon to the egg mixture and pour over the vegetables.
7. Sprinkle over the mozzarella cheese and dust with the paprika.
8. Bake for 25–35 minutes until bubbling and lightly browned.

Nutritional values per	Fat	Protein	Net Carbs
1 serving	27 g	19 g	9 g

Chicken stir-fry

Flexitarian friendly

Serves 6

2 Tbsp lemon juice
1 tsp xylitol
1 Tbsp Worcestershire sauce
¼ cup Banting tomato sauce (see recipe on page 130)
4 chicken breast fillets, cut into strips
1 Tbsp olive oil
1 medium onion, thinly sliced
1 medium green or red pepper, deseeded and thinly sliced
1 cm fresh ginger, peeled and grated
3 medium carrots, peeled and julienned
3 medium baby marrows, julienned
1 cup shredded cabbage
2 Tbsp water
salt and freshly ground black pepper to taste

1. Combine the lemon juice, xylitol, Worcestershire sauce and tomato sauce and use to marinade the chicken strips for 20 minutes.
2. Heat the oil in a frying pan and stir-fry the chicken in batches. Set aside the cooked chicken and keep the marinade.
3. In the same pan, fry the onion, green or red pepper and ginger for a few minutes.
4. Add the carrots and baby marrows, and fry until the vegetables are almost cooked, but not too soft.
5. Stir the cabbage, chicken strips and reserved marinade into the vegetables, add the water and cover with a lid. Simmer for a few minutes until the cabbage is just cooked.
6. Season to taste and serve warm.

Nutritional values per	Fat	Protein	Net Carbs
1 serving	16 g	26 g	8 g

Liza's fish tart

Flexitarian friendly

Serves 6

2 x 120 g cans sardines in brine
2 medium onions, chopped
1 medium red pepper, deseeded and chopped
1 tsp coconut oil
250 g mushrooms, chopped
salt and freshly ground black pepper to taste
4 large eggs, whisked
200 ml Greek yoghurt
1 cup grated Cheddar cheese

1. Preheat the oven to 180 °C.
2. Drain the sardines, fold them open and place them in the bottom of a casserole dish.
3. Lightly sauté the onions and red pepper in the coconut oil and place on top of the fish.
4. Top with the mushrooms and season with salt and pepper.
5. Mix the eggs and Greek yoghurt and pour over the mushrooms.
6. Top with the grated cheese.
7. Bake for 40 minutes or until cooked.

Nutritional values per	Fat	Protein	Net Carbs
1 serving	16 g	20 g	9 g

Crustless vegetable quiche

Lacto-ovo-vegetarian friendly

Serves 4

2 tsp olive oil
2 medium onions, chopped
3 medium baby marrows, sliced

4 large fresh spinach leaves, chopped
½ tsp salt
lemon juice and freshly ground black pepper to taste
3 large eggs
1 cup full-fat milk
1 tsp paprika
2 Tbsp chopped fresh parsley
¼ cup grated Cheddar cheese

1. Preheat the oven to 180 °C and grease a medium quiche or pie dish with butter.
2. Heat the oil in a frying pan and fry the onions and baby marrows for a few minutes.
3. Stir in the spinach and cook until soft.
4. Add the salt and season with lemon juice and black pepper.
5. Beat the eggs and milk with an electric beater and add the paprika and parsley.
6. Tip the vegetables into the greased dish and pour over the egg mixture.
7. Sprinkle the grated cheese evenly over the top.
8. Bake for 30–45 minutes until cooked.

Nutritional values per	Fat	Protein	Net Carbs
1 serving	13 g	11 g	9 g

DINNER

Beef curry bake

Serves 6

1 Tbsp coconut oil
1 medium onion, chopped

2 cups chopped mushrooms
500 g beef mince
115 g tomato paste
1 Tbsp apple cider vinegar
1 Tbsp xylitol
1 tsp crushed garlic
2 Tbsp mild curry powder
300 g mixed vegetables (try green beans, carrots and broccoli), chopped
4 eggs, whisked
1 cup full-fat milk
salt and freshly ground black pepper to taste
2 cups grated Cheddar cheese

1. Preheat the oven to 180 °C and grease a large ovenproof dish.
2. Melt the coconut oil in a large saucepan.
3. Lightly fry the onion, then add the mushrooms and fry until just cooked.
4. Add the mince and fry until browned.
5. Mix the tomato paste, apple cider vinegar, xylitol, garlic and curry powder and add to the mince.
6. Add the mixed vegetables and simmer until the mince is cooked and the vegetables are half-cooked. Spoon the mixture into the greased dish.
7. Combine the whisked eggs, milk, salt and pepper with 1½ cups of the grated cheese.
8. Pour this egg mixture over the mince and vegetables and top with the remaining grated cheese.
9. Bake for 45–55 minutes until the egg topping is set and the cheese is golden brown.
10. Serve warm with a side salad.

Nutritional values per	Fat	Protein	Net Carbs
1 serving	32 g	34 g	11 g

Greek chicken

Flexitarian friendly

Serves 4

50 ml butter
25 ml olive oil
8 chicken drumsticks, skin on
1 medium onion, finely chopped
1 clove garlic, crushed
1 Tbsp Banting Dijon mustard (see recipe on page 132)
50 ml tomato paste
50 ml water
3 medium tomatoes, peeled and chopped
juice of ½ lemon
1 tsp ground cinnamon
½ tsp dried origanum
salt and freshly ground black pepper to taste

1. Heat the butter and oil in a frying pan and fry the chicken drumsticks until lightly browned. Remove the chicken and set aside.
2. Add all the remaining ingredients to the pan and simmer for 10 minutes.
3. Add the chicken and simmer for a further 40 minutes.
4. Serve warm with either cauli rice (see recipe on page 124) or zucchini (baby marrow) noodles.

Nutritional values per	Fat	Protein	Net Carbs
1 serving	44 g	50 g	8 g

Banting burgers

Serves 4

Burger patties
500 g beef mince
1 small onion, grated
1 small tomato, grated
1 large egg, beaten
salt and freshly ground black pepper to taste
1 Tbsp apple cider vinegar
1 Tbsp chopped fresh coriander
1 Tbsp chopped fresh parsley
1 Tbsp Worcestershire sauce
25 ml Heba, plus extra for coating
¼ tsp ground cloves

To serve
4 large portobello mushrooms
2 Tbsp coconut oil
¼ cup full-fat cream cheese
8 cherry tomatoes, halved
120 g Cheddar cheese, grated

1. Preheat the oven to 180 °C.
2. Combine all the ingredients for the burger patties and divide the mixture in four.
3. Shape into four patties and coat each in extra Heba. Gently shake off the excess.
4. Place the mushrooms on a baking tray and grill in the oven for 20 minutes or until soft.
5. In the meantime, fry the patties in the coconut oil over medium heat until browned and cooked through.

6. Spread each grilled mushroom with a tablespoon of cream cheese and top with a burger patty.
7. Top each burger with cherry tomato halves and grated cheese, and season with salt and pepper if desired.
5. Grill the burgers in the oven until the cheese is nicely melted.
8. Serve immediately with a small side salad.

Nutritional values per	Fat	Protein	Net Carbs
1 serving	42 g	38 g	8 g

Trout with almonds

| Flexitarian friendly |

Serves 4

4 x 159 g trout fillets
salt and lemon juice to taste
200 ml chopped raw almonds
lemon slices and fresh parsley to garnish

1. Clean the fish fillets and dry them well.
2. Flavour the fish with salt and lemon juice.
3. Place the fish fillets in a frying pan and sprinkle over the almonds. Cover with a lid and allow the fish to simmer over a high heat for just a few minutes.
4. Keeping the lid on, turn down the heat and simmer for a further 15–20 minutes.
5. Serve immediately, garnished with lemon slices and fresh parsley.

Nutritional values per	Fat	Protein	Net Carbs
1 serving	31 g	33 g	5 g

Masala lamb chops

Eastern friendly

Serves 1

1 lamb loin chop

Marinade (per loin chop)

½ Tbsp Greek yoghurt
½ tsp lemon juice
½ tsp masala
½ tsp ground ginger
½ tsp tomato purée
salt to taste

1. Mix the marinade ingredients and use to coat the lamb chop.
2. Fry, grill or bake the chop as preferred.

Nutritional values per	Fat	Protein	Net Carbs
1 serving	32 g	16 g	2 g

Spinach and mushroom lasagne

Lacto-ovo-vegetarian friendly

Serves 4

2 Tbsp olive oil
1 onion, chopped
1 tsp crushed garlic
2 bunches fresh spinach, washed and chopped
salt to taste
1 onion, sliced
1 green pepper, deseeded and sliced
250 g mushrooms, sliced

freshly ground black pepper and dried origanum to taste
1 cup fresh cream
125 g full-fat cream cheese
½ tsp paprika
1 cup grated Cheddar cheese
garlic salt to taste

1. Heat half the oil in a saucepan and fry the chopped onion and garlic for a few minutes. Add the spinach and fry until soft. Drain any excess water and season with salt.
2. Heat the remaining oil in a frying pan and sauté the sliced onion and green pepper for a few minutes, then add the mushrooms. Season with salt and cook until all the water has evaporated. Remove from the heat and season with black pepper and dried origanum.
3. Preheat the oven to 180 °C.
4. Heat the cream and cream cheese in a small saucepan and mix until smooth. Stir in the paprika and half the grated cheese and season to taste with garlic salt, black pepper and dried origanum. Remove from the heat once the cheese has melted and the sauce is smooth.
5. Layer half the spinach on the bottom of an ovenproof dish, followed by the mushroom filling. Cover with the remaining spinach and pour over the cheese sauce. Top with the remaining grated cheese, black pepper and origanum.
6. Bake for 40 minutes until golden.

Nutritional values per	Fat	Protein	Net Carbs
1 serving	44 g	11 g	11 g

Chutney chicken

Flexitarian friendly

Serves 4

1 Tbsp olive oil
1 cinnamon stick
1 onion, sliced
1 tsp ginger and garlic paste
4 chicken breasts, skin on
1 Tbsp masala
½ tsp ground cumin
salt to taste
1 cup water
1 x 410 g can chopped tomatoes
1 green pepper, deseeded and diced
2 bay leaves
chopped fresh coriander to garnish

1. Heat the oil in a frying pan, add the cinnamon stick and onion, and fry until the onion is browned.
2. Add the ginger and garlic paste along with the chicken breasts and fry for 10 minutes until the chicken is golden on all sides.
3. Add the masala and cumin and mix well. Season with salt and add the water.
4. Cook for 30 minutes.
5. Add the chopped tomatoes, green pepper and bay leaves.
6. Cook for a further 20 minutes and garnish with chopped fresh coriander before serving.

Nutritional values per	Fat	Protein	Net Carbs
1 serving	10 g	27 g	8 g

Roti

Makes 10

4 eggs
62 ml milk
¼ cup coconut flour
½ tsp baking powder
½ tsp chilli powder
½ tsp ground cumin
¼ tsp ground coriander
a pinch of salt

1. Mix all the ingredients in a blender.
2. Heat a non-stick frying pan over medium heat and grease with a little ghee or coconut oil.
3. Pour a ladleful of batter into the pan and allow it to spread thinly by gently tilting the pan.
4. Cook for 3–4 minutes until small bubbles form on top, then flip the roti to cook the other side.

Nutritional values per	Fat	Protein	Net Carbs
1 serving	3 g	3 g	1 g

Aubergine curry

Serves 6

1 Tbsp olive oil
1 large onion, chopped
10 curry leaves
1 tsp crushed garlic
1 Tbsp masala

½ tsp ground turmeric

8 small aubergines, halved

salt to taste

½ cup water

6 tomatoes, grated

1 Tbsp tomato paste

1 tsp tamarind concentrate dissolved in ¼ cup water

chopped fresh coriander to garnish

1. Heat the oil in a large saucepan and fry the onion and curry leaves until the onion is transparent.
2. Add the garlic, masala, turmeric and aubergines and fry for 3–5 minutes.
3. Season with salt, add the water and cook for 10 minutes, taking care that it does not cook dry. Add more water if necessary.
4. Add the tomatoes and tomato paste and cook for a further 10 minutes.
5. Add the tamarind and cook for 5 minutes.
6. Garnish with chopped fresh coriander before serving.

Nutritional values per	Fat	Protein	Net Carbs
1 serving	21 g	23 g	9 g

Lamb curry with calabash

Eastern friendly

Serves 6

2 Tbsp olive oil

3 cinnamon sticks

2 star anise

2 bay leaves

10 curry leaves
1 onion, sliced
1 kg cubed lamb pieces
2 tsp ginger and garlic paste
1 Tbsp masala
1 tsp ground cumin
1 tsp ground coriander
¼ tsp ground turmeric
salt to taste
2 tomatoes, diced
1 cup water
1 large calabash, peeled and cut into chunks
chopped fresh coriander to garnish

1. Heat the oil in a large saucepan and add the cinnamon sticks, star anise, bay leaves, curry leaves and onion. Fry until the onion is browned.
2. Add the lamb and ginger and garlic paste. Fry for 10 minutes until the meat is well sealed.
3. Add the masala, cumin, coriander and turmeric and mix well.
4. Season with salt and then add the tomatoes and water.
5. Cook for 20 minutes.
6. Add the calabash and cook for a further 25 minutes or until the calabash is cooked.
7. Garnish with chopped fresh coriander to serve.

Nutritional values per	Fat	Protein	Net Carbs
1 serving	9 g	35 g	6 g

Fish cakes

Serves 8

100 g sweet potato, peeled and diced
1 onion, chopped
2–3 green chillies, chopped and deseeded if preferred
½ bunch fresh coriander, roughly chopped
600 g hake fillets, skinned and cubed
1 Tbsp crushed garlic
½ tsp curry powder
1 tsp ground cumin
1 tsp ground coriander
1 tsp garam masala
½ tsp chilli flakes
1 egg
salt to taste

1. Place the sweet potato in a microwaveable bowl with 2 cm water and microwave on high for 3 minutes or until cooked.
2. In a food processor, blitz the onion, chillies and fresh coriander.
3. Add the remaining ingredients, including the sweet potato, and pulse until the fish has broken up.
4. Roll the mixture into little balls between your palms. Flatten and shape the balls into fish cakes.
5. Shallow-fry the fish cakes in coconut oil over low–medium heat for about 4 minutes on each side or until cooked through.
6. Serve hot with the following double-cream yoghurt dip.

Double-cream yoghurt dip

1 cup double-thick yoghurt
1 Tbsp lemon juice
freshly ground black pepper, garlic salt and dried mixed herbs to taste

1. Combine all the ingredients and serve with the fish cakes.

Nutritional values per	Fat	Protein	Net Carbs
1 serving	5 g	15 g	4 g

Prawn korma

Flexitarian friendly
Eastern friendly

Serves 4

20 large king prawns, deveined
3 Tbsp plain yoghurt
45 g crème fraiche
1 tsp paprika
1 tsp garam masala
1 Tbsp tomato purée
1 Tbsp coconut milk
1 tsp chilli powder
½ cup water
1 Tbsp olive oil
1 tsp crushed garlic
1 cinnamon stick
½ tsp ground cardamom
salt to taste
chopped fresh coriander to garnish

1. Wash and drain the prawns, then pat dry, ensuring all the liquid is removed.
2. Place the yoghurt, crème fraiche, paprika, garam masala, tomato purée, coconut milk, chilli powder and water in a mixing bowl. Blend and set aside.
3. Heat the oil in a heavy-based frying pan and add the garlic, cinnamon stick, cardamom and salt to taste.

4. Turn up the heat and pour in the yoghurt-spice mixture. Bring to the boil, stirring occasionally.
5. Add the prawns and continue to cook for about 15 minutes until the sauce is thick.
6. Serve garnished with chopped fresh coriander.

Nutritional values per	Fat	Protein	Net Carbs
1 serving	10 g	5 g	3 g

Mince-stuffed peppers

Eastern friendly

Serves 4

4 green peppers
1 Tbsp olive oil
1 onion, chopped
1 tsp crushed ginger
1 tsp crushed garlic
1 Tbsp masala
400 g lamb mince
salt to taste
1 cup chopped green beans
1 tomato, grated
1 cup grated Cheddar cheese

1. Cut off the tops of the green peppers and scoop out the seeds and veins.
2. Bring a saucepan of water to the boil and add the peppers. Allow to cook and soften for 5 minutes, then drain in a colander.
3. Heat the oil in a frying pan and sauté the onion. Add the ginger, garlic and masala. Stir and add the mince.

4. Season with salt and cook for 20 minutes.
5. Add the green beans and tomato and simmer for 10 minutes.
6. Preheat the oven to 200 °C and grease a baking tray.
7. Fill the peppers with the mince mixture and sprinkle some grated cheese on top of each.
8. Place the stuffed peppers on the greased tray and cook for 20 minutes until the cheese is melted and golden.

Nutritional values per	Fat	Protein	Net Carbs
1 serving	34 g	29 g	11 g

Braised chicken livers

Flexitarian friendly
Eastern friendly

Serves 4

2 Tbsp coconut oil
1 large onion, chopped
1 Tbsp chopped garlic
2 red chillies, chopped
1 kg chicken livers
1 x 410 g can chopped peeled tomatoes
½ cup water
salt to taste

1. Heat the oil in a large frying pan and sauté the onion, garlic and chillies.
2. Add the chicken livers and fry until browned.
3. Add the tomatoes, water and salt to taste and simmer for 20 minutes.

Note: This dish is suitable for freezing.

Nutritional values per	Fat	Protein	Net Carbs
1 serving	13 g	23 g	6 g

Mutton stew

Traditional South African recipe

Serves 6

2 Tbsp olive oil

1 onion, diced

2 cloves garlic, crushed

1 kg stewing mutton

2 large aubergines, peeled and cubed

1 leek, thinly sliced (optional)

2 Tbsp chopped fresh marjoram

2 cups mutton or beef stock

1 red chilli, thinly sliced

chopped fresh rosemary and thyme to taste

salt and freshly ground black pepper to taste

1. Heat the oil in a large saucepan and lightly brown the onion and garlic.
2. Add the mutton, aubergines, leek (if using), marjoram, stock and chilli.
3. Add rosemary and thyme to taste, and season well with salt and pepper.
4. Cook for 1½ hours or until the meat is soft and succulent.
5. Serve with morogo (see recipe on page 123) and Heba pap (see recipe on page 95).

Nutritional values per	Fat	Protein	Net Carbs
1 serving	41 g	34 g	11 g

Sheep's liver in tomato jus

Traditional South African recipe

Serves 4

¼ cup olive oil

1 large onion, thinly sliced

2 cloves garlic, thinly sliced

2 Tbsp dried Italian herbs

1 cup water

4 large ripe tomatoes, thinly sliced

1 x 70 g can tomato paste

3 Tbsp Banting tomato sauce (see recipe on page 130)

salt and freshly ground black pepper to taste

500 g sheep's liver

2 Tbsp dried thyme

1. Heat half the oil in a frying pan and sauté the onion and garlic.
2. Add the dried Italian herbs and slowly increase the heat.
3. Add the water, tomatoes, tomato paste and tomato sauce and simmer for 10 minutes.
4. Season well with salt and pepper and simmer for a further 5 minutes.
5. Clean the liver and remove any hard tissue. Cut into thin strips and season with the dried thyme, salt and pepper.
6. Heat the remaining oil in a separate frying pan and slowly fry the liver strips for 4 minutes on each side.
7. Pour in the tomato jus and simmer for 5 minutes, stirring occasionally.
8. Serve warm with Heba pap (see recipe on page 95).

Nutritional values per	Fat	Protein	Net Carbs
1 serving	17 g	29 g	15 g

Tripe in tomato sauce

Serves 4

1.5 kg tripe
1 tsp salt
1 Tbsp lemon juice
¼ cup coconut oil
1 onion, finely chopped
2 carrots, peeled and diced
2 stalks celery, finely chopped
1 x 115 g can tomato paste
1 x 410 g can chopped peeled tomatoes
1 cup dry white wine
2 Tbsp xylitol

1. Wash and rinse the tripe thoroughly.
2. Place the tripe in a saucepan of cold water, add the salt and lemon juice, and bring to the boil. Reduce the heat and simmer gently for 2 hours or until tender. Drain, cut into cubes and set aside.
3. Heat the oil in a separate saucepan and add the remaining ingredients.
4. Simmer for 15 minutes and then add the parboiled tripe.
5. Cook for a further 20 minutes.
6. Serve hot with Heba pap (see recipe on page 95).

Nutritional values per	Fat	Protein	Net Carbs
1 serving	27 g	48 g	9 g

SIDES

Asparagus with tzatziki

Serves 6

200 g asparagus tips
½ cup Greek yoghurt
¼ cucumber, grated
2 cloves garlic, crushed
½ tsp ground coriander
salt and freshly ground black pepper to taste

1. Steam the asparagus until cooked.
2. Mix the yoghurt, cucumber, garlic, coriander, salt and pepper to make a tzatziki dip.
3. Serve the asparagus either hot or cold with the tzatziki.

Nutritional values per	Fat	Protein	Net Carbs
1 serving	1 g	2 g	3 g

Vegetable sosaties

Makes 24

1 large red onion, chopped into chunks
100 g patty pans
100 g red pepper, deseeded and chopped into chunks
100 g baby marrow, sliced into chunks
100 g butternut, peeled and chopped into chunks
100 g sweet potato, peeled and chopped into chunks
2 tsp olive oil
4 tsp white balsamic vinegar
½ tsp salt

freshly ground black pepper to taste
10 g fresh rosemary, chopped
10 g fresh thyme, chopped
24 sosatie sticks

1. Preheat the oven to 180 °C.
2. Place all the vegetables on a baking tray and drizzle with the olive oil and balsamic vinegar. Season with the salt, pepper, rosemary and thyme.
3. Roast the vegetables for about 30 minutes until cooked.
4. Thread one chunk of each vegetable onto a sosatie stick, repeating until you have 24 sosaties.
5. Serve with your choice of protein and a tzatziki dip (see recipe on page 120).

Nutritional values per	Fat	Protein	Net Carbs
1 serving	0 g	0 g	2 g

Broccoli cheese bake

Serves 4

1 medium-head broccoli, chopped
1 quantity Banting cheese sauce (see recipe on page 133)
1 cup grated Cheddar cheese

1. Preheat the oven to 180 °C.
2. Steam the broccoli until 90 per cent cooked. Drain and set aside.
3. Prepare the Banting cheese sauce as per the recipe on page 133.
4. Place the broccoli in a casserole dish, pour over the cheese sauce and top with the grated cheese.

5. Bake for 10–15 minutes or until the cheese is golden brown. Serve warm.

Nutritional values per	Fat	Protein	Net Carbs
1 serving	40 g	21 g	11 g

Crumbed aubergine

Serves 8

4 medium aubergines, peeled and sliced into thumb-size strips
salt for rubbing
2 large eggs, whisked
1 cup Heba
2 Tbsp coconut oil

1. Rub the aubergine strips with salt and stack them on top of each other. Cover with a plate and leave them as is for about 2 hours.
2. Pat dry the aubergine strips with paper towel, then dip them first in the whisked egg and then in the Heba to coat.
3. Heat the oil in a frying pan and fry the aubergine strips for 90 seconds on each side until cooked through and crispy.
4. Serve warm with a tzatziki dip (see recipe on page 120) or Banting mayonnaise (see recipe on page 129).

Nutritional values per	Fat	Protein	Net Carbs
1 serving	12 g	11 g	9 g

Morogo

Traditional African recipe

Serves 2

1 Tbsp butter
1 large onion, chopped
1 star anise
1 large bunch fresh morogo (wild spinach)
1 cup water
salt and freshly ground black pepper to taste
2 medium tomatoes, diced
2 Tbsp dried basil

1. Melt the butter in a saucepan and fry the onion until softened.
2. Add the star anise, morogo and water and season well with salt and pepper.
3. Allow to simmer until the leaves are soft.
4. Add the tomatoes and basil and simmer for a further 5–10 minutes.

Nutritional values per	Fat	Protein	Net Carbs
1 serving	8 g	10 g	13 g

Mayo-free coleslaw

Serves 30

6 cups thinly sliced cabbage
1 cup grated carrot
1 large red pepper, deseeded and sliced into thin strips
½ cup chopped fresh mint
½ cup chopped fresh coriander
10 red spring onions, thinly sliced

7 Tbsp apple cider vinegar

2 tsp sesame oil

2 tsp olive oil

salt and freshly ground black pepper to taste

chopped fresh coriander and sesame seeds to garnish

1. Mix the cabbage, carrot, red pepper, mint, coriander and spring onions in a large bowl.
2. Whisk the vinegar, sesame oil and olive oil in a small bowl and season to taste.
3. Drizzle the dressing over the salad and toss well.
4. Serve with some chopped coriander and sesame seeds scattered on top of each helping.

Nutritional values per	Fat	Protein	Net Carbs
1 serving	1 g	1 g	1 g

Cauli rice

Serves 4

1 onion, finely chopped

2 Tbsp butter

1 medium-head cauliflower

salt to taste

1. Sauté the onion in 1 Tbsp butter in a frying pan until soft.
2. Break the cauliflower into florets and microwave or steam until slightly soft (they must still be firm).
3. Pulse the cauliflower in a food processor to obtain the desired texture.
4. Add the onion and remaining butter and mix well. Season with salt to taste.

Nutritional values per	Fat	Protein	Net Carbs
1 serving	4 g	3 g	6 g

Cauli mash

Serves 4

2 medium-head cauliflowers
200 g full-fat cream cheese (optional)
2 Tbsp grated Parmesan cheese (optional)
a pinch of paprika
salt to taste

1. Steam or microwave the cauliflower until soft. Drain off the excess water.
2. Place the cauliflower in a food processor, add the remaining ingredients and blitz. Alternatively, use a hand-held stick blender.

Nutritional values per	Fat	Protein	Net Carbs
1 serving	20 g	10 g	12 g

Side salad

Serves 1

1 cup shredded lettuce
4 cherry tomatoes
¼ cup chopped cucumber
1 Tbsp chopped spring onion
3–5 olives
¼ round feta, crumbled
1 Tbsp olive oil

1 tsp balsamic vinegar

salt and freshly ground black pepper to taste

1. Combine all the ingredients in a bowl.

Nutritional values per	Fat	Protein	Net Carbs
1 serving	21 g	4 g	7 g

Cheese salad

To the above side salad, add:

30 g Cheddar cheese, cubed

an additional ¼ round feta, crumbled

½ medium avocado, cubed

Nutritional values per	Fat	Protein	Net Carbs
1 serving	47 g	16 g	10 g

Tomato soup

Serves 4

675 g tomatoes, chopped

4 spring onions, chopped

2 medium sweet red peppers, deseeded and chopped

1 tsp chopped garlic

salt and freshly ground black pepper to taste

1 bay leaf

1 Tbsp olive oil

3 cups water

2 Tbsp chopped fresh coriander

1. Preheat the oven to 200 °C.
2. Layer the tomatoes, spring onions, red peppers and garlic on a baking tray. Season with salt and pepper, add the bay leaf and drizzle over the olive oil. Roast the vegetables for 30 minutes or until softened and beginning to brown.
3. Bring the water to the boil in a saucepan and add the roasted vegetable mixture. Stir well and then blend in a food processor or with a hand-held stick blender until smooth.
4. Serve garnished with the chopped fresh coriander.

Nutritional values per	Fat	Protein	Net Carbs
1 serving	3 g	3 g	10 g

MISCELLANEOUS

Bone broth

Makes about 1.5 litres

1 kg bones (use beef, sheep, pig or chicken bones, or a combination)
4 medium carrots, roughly chopped
4 medium leeks, roughly chopped
a bunch of celery (leaves only), roughly chopped
2 bay leaves
2 Tbsp apple cider vinegar
1 Tbsp whole peppercorns
1 Tbsp natural salt

1. Preheat the oven to 200 °C and place the bones in a single layer on a baking tray.
2. Roast the bones for 30–60 minutes until browned (this is not essential, but adds to the flavour).

3. Add the bones and all the remaining ingredients to a slow cooker and add enough water to cover. You can cook the broth on the stove top, but most people are wary about leaving the stove on overnight.

4. Simmer on low for 24 hours. For the first few hours, try to skim off any impurities (foam/scum) that float to the surface and top up with water to keep the ingredients covered. The broth is done when it's deep brown in colour and deeply flavourful.

5. Once cooked, strain the broth through a fine-mesh sieve. Allow the clear liquid to cool to room temperature and then refrigerate. The broth should form a gel when cold, but will liquefy when heated.

Note: This broth can be stored in the refrigerator for up to five days and in the freezer for up to six months. A handy tip: Pour the bone broth into ice trays. One cube is just the right size in a coffee cup of hot water.

Brilliant Banting bread

Makes 1 loaf (about 15 slices)

1 cup almond flour
1 cup mixed seeds (100 g flax/100 g sunflower/50 g pumpkin)
¼ cup psyllium husk
1 tsp salt
2 tsp baking powder
6 eggs, beaten
1 cup Greek yoghurt

1. Preheat the oven to 140 °C and grease a standard loaf tin with butter.

2. Combine all the dry ingredients.
3. Add the beaten egg and mix well.
4. Stir in the yoghurt and pour the batter into the loaf tin.
5. Bake for 2 hours.

Nutritional values per	Fat	Protein	Net Carbs
1 slice	17 g	10 g	7 g

Banting salad dressing

Makes 300 ml

¼ cup apple cider vinegar
200 ml extra-virgin olive oil
2 Tbsp lemon juice
1 tsp crushed garlic
2 Tbsp chopped fresh herbs (any kind)
2 spring onions, finely chopped

1. Blend the ingredients.
2. Store in the fridge to keep the dressing fresh.

Note: This will keep in the fridge for up to two weeks.

Nutritional values per	Fat	Protein	Net Carbs
5 ml	3 g	0 g	0 g

Banting mayonnaise

Makes 250 ml

2 eggs
½ tsp mustard powder

½ tsp salt
2 tsp lemon juice
1 Tbsp white wine vinegar
1 cup avocado oil

1. Place the eggs, mustard, salt, lemon juice and vinegar in a blender.
2. Blend on medium speed until all the ingredients are mixed, and then slowly drizzle in the oil.
3. Continue to blend on low speed until all the oil is mixed in and the mayonnaise has thickened.
4. Store in a sealed, sterilised jar in the fridge.

Note: This will keep in the fridge for up to a week.

Nutritional values per	Fat	Protein	Net Carbs
5 ml	5 g	0 g	0 g

Banting tomato sauce

Makes 500 ml

100 ml extra-virgin olive oil
1 onion, chopped
1 stalk celery, chopped
½ cup grated pumpkin
1 tsp salt, or to taste
½ tsp freshly ground black pepper
2 cloves garlic, chopped
2 Tbsp unsalted butter
50 ml apple cider vinegar
2 x 410 g cans chopped peeled tomatoes
½ tsp ground allspice

2 bay leaves

3 Tbsp xylitol

1. Heat the oil in a large saucepan over medium heat.
2. Add the onion and cook until sweating.
3. Add the celery and pumpkin and season with the salt and pepper.
4. Sauté until all the vegetables are soft.
5. Add the garlic, butter and apple cider vinegar and cook for another 2 minutes.
6. Add the tomatoes, allspice, bay leaves and xylitol and simmer, covered, over low heat for 1 hour.
7. Remove the bay leaves and blend the tomato mixture until smooth.
8. Taste for seasoning.
9. Pour into a sterilised glass jar and allow to cool before sealing.

Note: This will keep in a sealed jar in the fridge for up to two weeks.

Nutritional values per	Fat	Protein	Net Carbs
5 ml	1 g	0 g	0 g

Banting cheeky chutney

Makes 500 ml

24 tomatoes

2 large onions

6 cloves garlic

6 red chillies

½ tsp paprika

1 Tbsp fresh ground ginger

2 Tbsp lime juice

1 Tbsp chopped fresh mint leaves
600 ml vinegar
1 cup xylitol
1 Tbsp salt

1. Blanche and peel the tomatoes.
2. Blend all the ingredients together in a food processor until as chunky or as smooth as you prefer.
3. Boil in a saucepan over low heat until thick and dark – usually a couple of hours.
4. Store in a sealed, sterilised glass jar.

Note: This will keep in a sealed jar in the fridge for up to two weeks.

Nutritional values per	Fat	Protein	Net Carbs
5 ml	0 g	0 g	2 g

Banting Dijon mustard

Makes 30 ml

1 Tbsp mustard powder
1 tsp water
1 tsp white wine vinegar, or ½ tsp white wine vinegar and ½ tsp white vinegar
1 Tbsp Banting mayonnaise (see recipe on page 129)
a pinch of xylitol

1. Combine all the ingredients and use immediately.

Nutritional values per	Fat	Protein	Net Carbs
30 ml	20 g	1 g	2 g
15 ml	10 g	1 g	1 g

Banting cheese sauce

Makes about 250 ml

1 Tbsp butter
½ cup cream
½ cup cream cheese
¼ tsp mustard powder
½ cup grated Cheddar cheese
salt to taste

1. Melt the butter in a saucepan and stir in the cream and cream cheese.
2. Add the mustard and grated cheese, and stir until the cheese has melted. Season with salt to taste.

Nutritional values per	Fat	Protein	Net Carbs
30 ml	14 g	5 g	2 g

Banting pepper sauce

Makes about 100 ml

3 Tbsp whole peppercorns
60 g butter
1 small onion, minced or finely grated
50 ml brandy
100 ml beef stock (homemade)
60 ml cream
salt to taste

1. Slightly crush the peppercorns, using either a mortar and pestle or a rolling pin.

2. Melt the butter in a saucepan over medium heat. Add the onion and sauté until soft.
3. Add the peppercorns and brandy and boil for 2 minutes, then add the beef stock and allow the mixture to reduce by half.
4. Add the cream and reduce until thickened. Season with salt to taste.

Note: If you are having pan-fried steak, the sauce can be made in the same pan using the meat drippings.

Nutritional values per	Fat	Protein	Net Carbs
30 ml	18 g	2 g	5 g

Banting mushroom sauce

Makes about 250 ml

1 Tbsp butter
½ onion, finely chopped
250 g mushrooms, finely chopped
1 cup cream
salt and pepper to taste

1. Melt the butter in a saucepan and fry the onion until soft.
2. Add the mushrooms and fry until light brown.
3. Slowly add the cream, allowing the sauce to reduce and thicken. Season to taste.

Nutritional values per	Fat	Protein	Net Carbs
30 ml	7 g	2 g	3 g

PART 7

MEAL PLANS

In this section we give you four meal plans to choose from. Meal Plan 1 is for 'profoundly insulin-resistant' Banters and nutritional ketosis; Meal Plan 2 is for those following a traditional African diet; Meal Plan 3 is for lacto-ovo-vegetarian and flexitarian Banters; and Meal Plan 4 is for those following a more Eastern diet.

- Please note that these meal plans are for women. For men, simply increase portion sizes for proteins and fats.
- Unless it specifically states 'raw', weights are for cooked food, so you will need to weigh the food once it's cooked, boiled, fried, grilled, etc. The reason we work mostly with cooked food is that most people don't eat their food raw and the minute you cook a portion of food, its nutritional value changes.
- The total macronutrient values will differ from day to day because we mix raw and cooked ingredients at meal times and that will influence the calculation of the macro values.
- The macronutrient values given are estimates only.
- If you can tolerate more carbs, you can increase your vegetable portions, add fruit (the low-carb options from the orange list) or include some orange-list proteins.
- If you are carb sensitive, stick to Meal Plan 1 or follow the days on the other meal plans that cater for less than 25 g net carbs.

- If you are sensitive to fat, reduce the amount of fat with which you cook, stick to the days with the least total fat or eat lean proteins instead of fatty meats, and rather include other healthy fats such as avocado and nuts.
- You may add spices or herbs to your meals (refer to the green list).
- You may have coffee or tea, preferably black with no sweetener. If you are going to include milk (2 tablespoons per cup) or cream (1 tablespoon per cup), remember to add those macronutrient values to the total macronutrient values for the day.
- Always start your day with a glass of water.
- If you want to know your unique macronutrient values of fats, proteins and carbs, contact us and we will calculate them for you. This is where we fine-tune for ultimate weight loss.

MEAL PLAN 1: FOR 'PROFOUNDLY INSULIN-RESISTANT' BANTERS AND NUTRITIONAL KETOSIS

Day 1

BREAKFAST
Ratatouille with eggs
1 serving ratatouille with eggs on 1 slice Banting toast
recipe on p. 89
Water

LUNCH
Salad with chicken strips
50 g lettuce
50 g tomato
50 g cucumber
30 g feta cheese
50 g cooked chicken strips (optional)
1 Tbsp extra-virgin olive oil, for dressing
Water

DINNER
Beef steak with cheese sauce and asparagus with tzatziki
100 g beef rump steak, grilled
2 Tbsp Banting cheese sauce *recipe on p. 133*
1 serving asparagus with tzatziki *recipe on p. 120*
Water

Estimated macronutrient values for the day (in grams)		
Fat	Protein	Net Carbs
83	76	25

Day 2

BREAKFAST
Cream-cheese pancakes
2 servings cream-cheese pancakes without topping *recipe on p. 96*
1 Tbsp whipped cream, for topping
Water

LUNCH
Salad with leftover beef steak
50 g lettuce
50 g tomato
50 g cucumber
30 g feta cheese
50 g leftover beef steak (optional)
Water

DINNER
Greek chicken with crumbled aubergine
1 serving Greek chicken *recipe on p. 104*
1 serving crumbled aubergine *recipe on p. 122*
Water

Estimated macronutrient values for the day (in grams)		
Fat	Protein	Net Carbs
112	87	23

Day 3

BREAKFAST
Bacon omelette
2 large eggs
50 g cured bacon, pan-fried/grilled
recipe on p. 92
Water

LUNCH
Liza's fish tart
1 serving Liza's fish tart
recipe on p. 101
Water

DINNER
Burger with salad
1 serving Banting burger *recipe on p. 105*
1 serving side salad *recipe on p. 125*
Water

Estimated macronutrient values for the day (in grams)		
Fat	Protein	Net Carbs
127	93	25

Day 4

BREAKFAST
Bacon and feta quiche
1 serving bacon and feta quiche
recipe on p. 92
Water

LUNCH
Chicken stir-fry
1 serving chicken stir-fry
recipe on p. 100
Water

DINNER
Lamb chop with vegetable sosaties
150 g lamb loin chop, grilled
2 vegetable sosaties
recipe on p. 120
Water

Estimated macronutrient values for the day (in grams)		
Fat	Protein	Net Carbs
99	86	25

Day 5

BREAKFAST
Boere breakfast
1 serving Heba pap *recipe on p. 95*
50 g beef boerewors, grilled
1 large egg, poached
Water

LUNCH
Salad only
50 g lettuce
50 g tomato
50 g cucumber
1 Tbsp extra-virgin olive oil, for dressing
Water

DINNER
Trout with almonds and broccoli cheese bake
1 serving trout with almonds *recipe on p. 106*
1 serving broccoli cheese bake *recipe on p. 121*
Water

Estimated macronutrient values for the day (in grams)		
Fat	Protein	Net Carbs
130	98	25

Day 6

BREAKFAST
Fried breakfast with cheese
1 large egg, scrambled
50 g cured bacon, pan-fried/grilled
50 g feta cheese
1 Tbsp butter, for cooking
Water

LUNCH
Cheese salad
1 serving cheese salad
recipe on p. 126
Water

DINNER
Beef curry bake with mayo-free coleslaw
1 serving beef curry bake *recipe on p. 102*
1 serving mayo-free coleslaw *recipe on p. 123*
Water

Estimated macronutrient values for the day (in grams)		
Fat	Protein	Net Carbs
119	75	23

Day 7

BREAKFAST
Quick egg muffins with cheese
2 servings quick egg muffins *recipe on p. 93*
30 g Gouda cheese
Water

LUNCH
Tomato soup with halloumi bites
1 serving tomato soup *recipe on p. 126*
50 g halloumi cheese, lightly fried in a non-stick pan
Water

DINNER
Pork chop with salad
150 g pork loin chop, grilled
50 g lettuce
50 g cucumber
30 g feta cheese
1 Tbsp extra-virgin olive oil, for dressing
Water

Estimated macronutrient values for the day (in grams)		
Fat	Protein	Net Carbs
100	82	21

MEAL PLAN 2: TRADITIONAL AFRICAN

Day 1

BREAKFAST

Fried eggs, mushrooms and tomato
2 large eggs, fried
50 g mushrooms, fried
50 g tomato, fried
1 Tbsp coconut oil, for frying
Water

LUNCH

Egg, tomato and lettuce sandwich
1 serving Heba bread in a mug
refer to package instructions
2 large eggs, fried
50 g tomato
50 g lettuce
Water

DINNER

Mutton stew with morogo and pap
1 serving mutton stew
recipe on p. 117
1 serving morogo
recipe on p. 123
1 serving side salad
recipe on p. 125
1 serving Heba pap
recipe on p. 95
Water

Fat	Protein	Net Carbs
121	84	36

Estimated macronutrient values for the day (in grams)

Day 2

BREAKFAST

Bacon, eggs and avocado
2 large eggs, fried
50 g cured bacon, pan-fried/grilled
50 g avocado
1 Tbsp coconut oil, for frying
Water

LUNCH

Tomato soup
1 serving tomato soup
recipe on p. 126
Water

DINNER

Sheep's liver in tomato jus with salad
1 serving sheep's liver in tomato jus
recipe on p. 118
1 serving side salad
recipe on p. 125
Water

Fat	Protein	Net Carbs
103	68	34

Estimated macronutrient values for the day (in grams)

Day 3

BREAKFAST

Pap and eggs
1 serving Heba pap
recipe on p. 95
2 large eggs, fried
1 Tbsp coconut oil, for frying
Water

LUNCH

Chicken salad
1 serving side salad
recipe on p. 125
50 g chicken strips, fried (optional)
1 Tbsp coconut oil, for frying
Water

DINNER

Tripe in tomato sauce
1 serving tripe in tomato sauce
recipe on p. 119
Water

Fat	Protein	Net Carbs
108	93	21

Estimated macronutrient values for the day (in grams)

Day 4

BREAKFAST

Chicken livers with cheese and tomato
100 g chicken livers, fried
50 g tomato
30 g Gouda cheese
1 Tbsp coconut oil, for frying
Water

LUNCH

Tuna salad
1 serving side salad
recipe on p. 125
100 g tuna
Water

DINNER

Chicken gizzards and giblets with morogo and salad
50 g chicken gizzards, fried
50 g chicken giblets, fried
1 Tbsp coconut oil, for frying
1 serving morogo
recipe on p. 123
1 serving side salad
recipe on p. 125
Water

Fat	Protein	Net Carbs
101	97	28

Estimated macronutrient values for the day (in grams)

Day 5

BREAKFAST

Eggs and morogo
2 large eggs, scrambled
1 serving morogo
recipe on p. 123
1 Tbsp coconut oil, for cooking
Water

LUNCH

Cheese salad
1 serving cheese salad
recipe on p. 126
Water

DINNER

Pork chop with roasted vegetables
150 g pork loin chop, grilled
50 g cauliflower, roasted
50 g carrot, roasted
50 g broccoli, steamed
1 Tbsp coconut oil, for roasting
Water

Fat	Protein	Net Carbs
119	81	29

Estimated macronutrient values for the day (in grams)

Day 6

BREAKFAST

Heba bread with eggs and mushrooms
1 serving Heba bread in a mug
refer to package instructions
2 large eggs, fried
100 g mushrooms, fried
1 Tbsp coconut oil, for frying
Water

LUNCH

Tomato soup with cheese
1 serving tomato soup
recipe on p. 126
30 g Gouda cheese, lightly fried
Water

DINNER

Hake with vegetables
150 g hake, fried
100 g green beans, steamed
½ cup gem squash, steamed
1 Tbsp butter, for gem squash
1 Tbsp coconut oil, for frying
Water

Fat	Protein	Net Carbs
85	71	23

Estimated macronutrient values for the day (in grams)

Day 7

BREAKFAST

Heba porridge and amasi with avocado
1 serving Heba porridge
recipe on p. 95
50 ml amasi
50 g avocado
Water

LUNCH

Pilchard salad
100 g canned pilchards in brine
1 serving side salad
recipe on p. 125
Water

DINNER

Braised chicken livers with pap
1 serving braised chicken livers
recipe on p. 116
1 serving Heba pap
recipe on p. 95
Water

Fat	Protein	Net Carbs
81	77	26

Estimated macronutrient values for the day (in grams)

MEAL PLAN 3: FOR LACTO-OVO-VEGETARIAN AND FLEXITARIAN BANTERS

Day 1

BREAKFAST
Toast with scrambled eggs and cheese
- 2 x 25 g slices grain-free toast (Life Bake)
- 2 large eggs, scrambled
- 30 g Cheddar cheese
- 1 Tbsp coconut oil, for cooking
- Water

LUNCH
Crustless vegetable quiche
- 1 serving crustless vegetable quiche *recipe on p. 101*
- Water

DINNER
Spinach and mushroom lasagne with salad
- 1 serving spinach and mushroom lasagne *recipe on p. 107*
- 1 serving spinach and mushroom salad
- 50 g lettuce
- 50 g tomato
- 30 g feta cheese
- 1 tsp Banting salad dressing *recipe on p. 129*
- Water

	Fat	Protein	Net Carbs
Estimated macronutrient values	113	58	28

Day 2

BREAKFAST
Ratatouille with eggs
- 1 serving ratatouille with eggs on 1 slice Banting toast *recipe on p. 128*
- Water

LUNCH
Mini eggs platter
- 2 large eggs, boiled
- 50 g tomato
- 30 g Gouda cheese
- Water

DINNER
Aubergine curry with cauli rice
- 1 serving aubergine curry *recipe on p. 110*
- 1 serving cauli rice *recipe on p. 124*
- Water

	Fat	Protein	Net Carbs
Estimated macronutrient values	71	66	35

Day 3

BREAKFAST
Spinach and feta omelette
- 2 large eggs
- 100 g baby-leaf spinach, boiled
- 30 g feta cheese
- 1 Tbsp coconut oil, for cooking
- Water

LUNCH
Crackers with cream cheese, tomato and cucumber
- 4 x 8 grain-free crackers (Life Bake)
- 50 g full-fat cream cheese
- 50 g tomato
- 50 g cucumber
- Water

DINNER
Roti with roasted vegetables and feta
- 50 g broccoli, roasted
- 50 g cauliflower, roasted
- 50 g baby marrow, roasted
- 50 g mushrooms, roasted
- 50 g green pepper, roasted
- 50 g red pepper, roasted
- 1 Tbsp coconut oil, for roasting
- 30 g feta cheese
- 1 serving roti *recipe on p. 110*
- Water

	Fat	Protein	Net Carbs
Estimated macronutrient values	86	47	18

Day 4

BREAKFAST
Herbed eggs and tomato on toast
- 1 serving herbed eggs and tomato on toast *recipe on p. 91*
- Water

LUNCH
Cheese salad with chicken strips
- 1 serving cheese salad *recipe on p. 126*
- 50 g cooked chicken breast strips
- Water

DINNER
Trout with almonds and mayo-free coleslaw
- 1 serving trout with almonds *recipe on p. 106*
- 1 serving mayo-free coleslaw *recipe on p. 123*
- Water

	Fat	Protein	Net Carbs
Estimated macronutrient values	107	99	31

Day 5

BREAKFAST
Cream-cheese pancakes with cheese
- 2 servings cream-cheese pancakes with topping *recipe on p. 96*
- Water

LUNCH
Chicken stir-fry with salad
- 1 serving chicken stir-fry *recipe on page 100*
- 50 g lettuce
- 50 g tomato
- 30 g feta cheese
- 50 g cucumber
- 1 tsp Banting salad dressing *recipe on p. 129*
- Water

DINNER
Fish cakes, asparagus with tzatziki and vegetable sosatie
- 1 serving fish cakes *recipe on p. 113*
- 1 serving asparagus with tzatziki *recipe on p. 120*
- 1 vegetable sosatie *recipe on p. 120*
- Water

	Fat	Protein	Net Carbs
Estimated macronutrient values	67	62	25

Day 6

BREAKFAST
Quick egg muffins with cheese
- 2 servings quick egg muffins *recipe on p. 93*
- 30 g Gouda cheese
- Water

LUNCH
Cheese salad
- 1 serving cheese salad *recipe on p. 126*
- Water

DINNER
Hake with broccoli cheese bake
- 150 g hake, steamed
- 1 serving broccoli cheese bake *recipe on p. 121*
- Water

	Fat	Protein	Net Carbs
Estimated macronutrient values	127	87	29

Day 7

BREAKFAST
Heba porridge with cinnamon and strawberries
- 1 serving Heba porridge *recipe on p. 95*
- 2 Tbsp full-cream milk, for porridge
- 1 tsp ground cinnamon
- 100 g strawberries
- Water

LUNCH
Liza's fish tart with salad
- 1 serving Liza's fish tart *recipe on p. 101*
- 50 g lettuce
- 50 g tomato
- 30 g feta cheese
- 50 g cucumber
- 1 Tbsp extra-virgin olive oil, for dressing
- Water

DINNER
Chutney chicken with cauli rice and salad
- 1 serving chutney chicken *recipe on p. 109*
- 1 serving cauli rice *recipe on p. 124*
- 50 g lettuce
- 50 g tomato
- 30 g feta cheese
- 50 g cucumber
- 1 Tbsp extra-virgin olive oil, for dressing
- Water

	Fat	Protein	Net Carbs
Estimated macronutrient values	91	63	32

MEAL PLAN 4: EASTERN

Day 1

BREAKFAST
Fried eggs with chicken sausage
2 large eggs, fried
1 chicken sausage, grilled
½ cup chopped mushrooms, fried
1 Tbsp butter, for frying
Water

LUNCH
Sardine salad on toast
1 x 120 g can sardines in brine
4 cherry tomatoes
½ cup chopped cucumber
1 cup shredded lettuce
1 Tbsp olive oil, for dressing
1 Tbsp balsamic vinegar, for dressing
1 x 25 g slice grain-free toast (Life Bake)
Water

DINNER
Masala lamb chops with vegetables
1 serving masala lamb chops
recipe on p. 107
½ cup cauli mash
1 serving side salad
recipe on p. 125
½ cup chopped pumpkin
½ cup chopped broccoli
Water

Fat	Protein	Net Carbs
104	86	26

Estimated macronutrient values

Day 2

BREAKFAST
Berry yoghurt smoothie
150 ml plain yoghurt
50 ml fresh cream
60 g raspberries
1 tsp xylitol (optional)
Blend all the ingredients together to make a smoothie
Water

LUNCH
Cheese salad
1 serving cheese salad
recipe on p. 126
1 Tbsp Banting salad dressing
recipe on p. 129
Water

DINNER
Spinach and mushroom lasagne with salad
1 serving spinach and mushroom lasagne
recipe on p. 107
1 serving side salad
recipe on p. 125
Water

Fat	Protein	Net Carbs
116	41	32

Estimated macronutrient values

Day 3

BREAKFAST
Stuffed mushrooms
1 large portobello mushroom
For the stuffing:
1 Tbsp finely chopped leek
½ tsp crushed garlic
28 g grated Cheddar cheese
1 tsp grated Parmesan cheese
1 Tbsp olive oil
Mix the stuffing ingredients, pile onto the mushroom and grill
Water

LUNCH
Tuna mayonnaise on toast
1 x 170 g can tuna in brine
1 pickled cucumber, chopped
1 cup shredded lettuce
½ green pepper
½ tomato, chopped
1 Tbsp Banting mayonnaise
recipe on p. 129
1 x 25 g slice grain-free toast (Life Bake)
Water

DINNER
Chutney chicken roti with salad
1 serving chutney chicken
recipe on p. 109
3 servings roti
recipe on p. 110
1 serving side salad
recipe on p. 125
Water

Fat	Protein	Net Carbs
90	79	22

Estimated macronutrient values

Day 4

BREAKFAST
Braised chicken livers
1 serving braised chicken livers
recipe on p. 116
1 serving Heba bread
refer to package instructions
1 Tbsp butter, for spreading
Water

LUNCH
Chutney eggs
Ingredients are enough for 3 servings, but have only 1 serving
Heat the following in a saucepan:
1 onion, chopped and fried in 1 Tbsp olive oil
1 tsp crushed garlic
2 red chillies, chopped
1 x 410 g can chopped, peeled tomatoes
1 Tbsp masala
Add 6 boiled eggs to the sauce
Water

DINNER
Mince-stuffed peppers with salad
1 serving mince-stuffed peppers
recipe on p. 115
1 serving side salad
recipe on p. 125
Water

Fat	Protein	Net Carbs
84	72	34

Estimated macronutrient values

Day 5

BREAKFAST
Chia-seed porridge
1 serving warm chia-seed porridge
recipe on p. 94
Water

LUNCH
Tomato soup with salad
1 serving tomato soup
recipe on p. 126
1 serving side salad
recipe on p. 125
Water

DINNER
Aubergine curry with cauli rice
1 serving aubergine curry
recipe on p. 110
½ cup cauli rice
recipe on p. 124
Water

Fat	Protein	Net Carbs
78	20	43

Estimated macronutrient values

Day 6

BREAKFAST
Vegetable omelette
Ingredients are enough for 2, but have only 1 serving
4 eggs, beaten with 2 Tbsp water
1 baby marrow, chopped
1 Tbsp finely chopped red pepper
½ cup chopped fresh spinach
1 small onion, chopped
1 small tomato, chopped
1 hot red chilli, chopped
season with ground turmeric and chopped fresh coriander
Water

LUNCH
Bunless burger with salad
120 g lamb mince seasoned with spice of your choice
Shape into patty and fry in a little oil
½ small onion, sliced into rings, fried in oil and 2 Tbsp balsamic vinegar
Serve with 1 Tbsp sour cream, 50 g avocado and 2 slices tomato
1 serving side salad
recipe on p. 125
Water

DINNER
Lamb curry with calabash
1 serving lamb curry with calabash
recipe on p. 111
½ cup cauli rice
recipe on p. 124
Water

Fat	Protein	Net Carbs
109	90	35

Estimated macronutrient values

Day 7

BREAKFAST
Cream-cheese pancakes
2 servings cream-cheese pancakes with topping
recipe on p. 96
Water

LUNCH
Fish cakes with salad
2 servings fish cakes
recipe on p. 113
1 serving side salad
recipe on p. 125
Water

DINNER
Prawn korma
1 serving prawn korma
recipe on p. 114
½ cup cauli rice
recipe on p. 124
Water

Fat	Protein	Net Carbs
66	36	20

Estimated macronutrient values

PART 8

FOOD LISTS AND INGREDIENTS LIST

The food lists are where we start to learn about what is healthy real food and what is not. Even though some real foods may seem healthy, it is good to remember that certain real foods, like potatoes and corn, are high in carbohydrates. These foods can raise insulin levels, which we now know results in fat accumulation. Below we explain how to read the food lists. Refer to the standard 'swap-out' list on page 35 when you want to quickly see which green-list products you can substitute for unhealthy products.

The lists

The Green Food List is the only list that you can eat from on a daily basis. These are the foods that are nutritious, low in carbs per portion and extremely healthy. Practising portion control is still important when eating from this list.

The Orange Food List is for people who have reached their goal weight and want to include some of the vegetables and berries on this list, or for those who are not sensitive to carbohydrates and can tolerate these vegetables and fruits. This list is also fine for an occasional sweet treat, but only once you have reached your goal weight.

The Red Food List must be avoided at all costs. We don't even recommend these foods as a once-in-a-while treat, as they are highly processed and contain unhealthy additives and chemicals.

The Yellow Food List contains the nutritional values of some other Banting-friendly products like grain-free toast and Heba pap/porridge. We've also included alcohol on the yellow list. You may only consume alcohol occasionally, and only what is listed here, nothing else.

The Ingredients List includes different names for soy and sugar. This list is to warn you of what to look out for on food labels.

How to read the food lists

1. Food/product: This is the description of the food or product and its form, whether cooked or raw.
2. Portion/serving size: These are our recommended serving sizes.
3. Macronutrients (fat/protein/glycaemic/net carbs): These are the macronutrient values for each portion/serving size. Some foods only contain fats and proteins, others only proteins and carbs, etc.
4. *LIND*: This sign indicates foods that are perfect for people who are 'profoundly insulin resistant' and for those who aim to achieve nutritional ketosis.

The Red Food List does not have portion/serving sizes or macro-nutrient values because ideally you are never going to eat or drink anything from this list. We have tried our best to indicate as many red food items as possible, but if you do come across a food or product that is not on the list, refer to the Ingredients List first to see if that can help you determine whether it's Banting friendly or not. If the product or food is not listed there, you are welcome to make contact with us through social media and we will try to help you.

Please note: The food lists have been compiled using the South African Food Data System and the USDA Food Composition Database. Portions given are based on females only. For men, portions may be increased on meat, dairy and vegetables.

GREEN FOOD LIST					
Food/product	Portion/ serving size	Fat (g)	Protein (g)	Glycaemic/ net carb (g)	*LIND* (low insulinogenic nutrient dense

REF: * raw weight / # cooked weight. If you are going to eat the food raw, weigh it and work on raw weight only; if you are going to cook the food, only weigh the food once cooked and work on cooked values.

PROTEINS					
Eggs					
Chicken, whole egg (boiled)#	1 x large (±51 g)	5.2	6.3	0.6	*LIND*
Chicken, whole egg (fried)#	1 x large	6.8	6.3	0.4	*LIND*
Chicken, whole egg (omelette)#	1 x large	7.11	6.5	0.4	*LIND*
Chicken, whole egg (poached)#	1 x large	4.7	6.3	0.4	*LIND*
Chicken, whole egg (scrambled)#	1 x large	6.7	6.1	1.0	*LIND*
Chicken, whole egg (scrambled)#	1 cup (220 g)	24.2	22	3.5	*LIND*
Beef					
Beef, biltong (cured, dried)	25 g	6.4	8.3	2.3	
Beef, boerewors (sausage, beef & pork) (grilled)#	150 g	54.5	20.7	4.1	*LIND*
Beef, brisket (cooked)#	100 g	28.4	22.1	0.0	
Beef, chuck (cooked)#	100 g	15.1	26.8	0.0	
Beef, droëwors	28 g	3.0	15.0	1.0	
Beef, fillet (cooked)#	100 g	7.5	30.9	0.0	
Beef, fore shin (cooked)#	100 g	6.2	30.6	0.0	
Beef, hind shin (cooked)#	100 g	14.3	28.9	0.0	
Beef, loin (cooked)#	100 g	16.6	29.0	0.0	
Beef, mince, regular (cooked)#	100 g	28.4	22.1	0.0	*LIND*
Beef, mince, lean (cooked)#	100 g	10.7	30.4	0.0	*LIND*
Beef, neck (cooked)#	100 g	18.8	26.7	0.0	
Beef, oxtail, meat only, salt added (stewed)#	100 g	13.4	30.5	0.0	
Beef, patty, frozen (grilled)#	100 g	21.8	23.1	0.3	
Beef, rib, prime (cooked)#	100 g	18.2	27.4	0.0	
Beef, rib, wing (cooked)#	100 g	16.5	28.6	0.0	
Beef, rump (cooked)#	100 g	17.0	29.2	0.0	*LIND*
Beef, shoulder (cooked)#	100 g	13.8	28.5	0.0	
Beef, silverside (cooked)#	100 g	9.1	30.7	0.0	
Beef, stock, homemade#	100 ml	0.1	2.0	1.2	
Beef, thick flank (cooked)#	100 g	7.5	31.5	0.0	
Beef, thin flank (cooked)#	100 g	22.0	24.0	0.0	
Beef, topside (cooked)#	100 g	10.7	30.4	0.0	
Chicken					
Chicken, dark meat, fresh (cooked – moist)#	100 g	9.7	25.5	0.0	*LIND*
Chicken, dark meat, frozen (cooked – moist)#1	100 g	5.3	28.4	0.0	*LIND*
Chicken, feet (raw)*	100 g	13.3	20.3	0.9	*LIND*
Chicken, meat & skin, frozen (roasted)*	100 g	13.0	25.6	0.0	*LIND*
Chicken, meat only, frozen (roasted)*	100 g	6.5	27.6	0.0	*LIND*
Chicken, stock, homemade#	100 ml	1.2	2.5	3.5	*LIND*
Chicken, white meat, fresh (cooked – moist)#2	100 g	4.1	28.6	0.0	*LIND*
Chicken, white meat, frozen (cooked – moist)#2	100 g	3.9	30.2	0.0	*LIND*
1 – dark meat includes drums & thighs 2 – white meat includes wings, breast & mince					
Duck					
Duck, meat & skin (roasted)#	150 g	42.6	28.5	0.0	*LIND*
Game					
Biltong, game	25 g	1.8	16.7	0.0	
Crocodile (cooked)#	100 g	8.2	30.9	0.0	

GREEN FOOD LIST

Food/product	Portion/ serving size	Fat (g)	Protein (g)	Glycaemic/ net carb (g)	*LIND* (low insulinogenic, nutrient dense)
Venison (buck/deer) (roasted)#	100 g	3.2	30.2	0.0	

Goat

Goat (roasted)#	100 g	3.0	27.1	0.0	

Goose

Goose, meat & skin (roasted)#	100 g	21.9	25.2	0.0	

Lamb/mutton

Lamb, cubed for stew (leg & shoulder) (braised)#	100 g	8.8	33.7	0.0	*LIND*
Lamb, leg, shank half (roasted)#	100 g	12.5	26.4	0.0	*LIND*
Lamb, leg, whole (shank & sirloin) (roasted)#	100 g	16.5	25.6	0.0	*LIND*
Lamb, loin chop (fast-fried)#	100 g	27.1	21.5	0.0	*LIND*
Lamb, neck chops (braised)#	100 g	21.4	28.5	0.0	*LIND*
Lamb, rack (fast-roasted)#	125 g	27.6	22.9	0.1	*LIND*
Lamb, rib (roasted)#	100 g	29.8	21.1	0.0	*LIND*
Mutton, leg, meat & fat (roasted)#	100 g	16.5	25.6	0.0	
Mutton, leg & shoulder, lean, meat only (braised)#	100 g	8.8	33.7	0.0	
Mutton, loin chop (grilled)#	100 g	23.1	25.2	0.0	
Mutton, mince (cooked)#	100 g	19.7	24.8	0.0	
Mutton, rib (grilled/roasted)#	100 g	29.8	21.1	0.2	
Mutton, rib, fat trimmed (grilled/roasted)#	100 g	29.6	22.1	0.1	
Mutton, shoulder (braised)#	100 g	24.6	28.7	0.0	

Organ meats (offal)

Beef, heart (simmered)#	100 g	4.7	28.5	0.2	*LIND*
Beef, kidney (simmered)#	100 g	4.7	27.3	0.0	*LIND*
Beef, liver (fried)#	100 g	4.7	26.5	5.2	*LIND*
Beef, lung (braised)#	100 g	3.7	20.4	0.0	*LIND*
Beef, pancreas (braised)#	100 g	17.2	27.1	0.0	*LIND*
Beef, spleen (braised)#	100 g	4.2	25.1	0.0	*LIND*
Beef, tongue (simmered)#	125 g	27.9	24.1	0.0	*LIND*
Beef, variety meats & by-products, tripe (simmered)#	200 g	8.2	23.4	4.0	*LIND*
Chicken, giblets (simmered)#	100 g	4.5	27.2	0.0	*LIND*
Chicken, gizzard, all classes (simmered)#	100 g	2.7	30.4	0.0	*LIND*
Chicken, heart, all classes (simmered)#	100 g	7.9	26.4	0.1	*LIND*
Chicken, liver (simmered)#	100 g	6.5	24.5	0.9	*LIND*
Lamb/sheep, brain (braised)#	200 g	20.4	25.2	0.4	*LIND*
Lamb/sheep, heart (braised)#	100 g	7.9	25.0	1.9	*LIND*
Lamb/sheep, kidney (braised)#	100 g	3.6	23.7	1.0	*LIND*
Lamb/sheep, liver (fried)#	100 g	12.7	25.5	3.8	*LIND*
Lamb/sheep, lung (braised)#	150 g	4.7	29.9	0.0	*LIND*
Lamb/sheep, pancreas (braised)#	100 g	15.1	22.8	0.3	*LIND*
Lamb/sheep, spleen (braised)#	100 g	4.8	26.5	0.4	*LIND*
Lamb/sheep, tongue (braised)#	100 g	20.3	21.6	0.0	*LIND*
Offal, tripe/brawn/brain/tongue (cooked)#	150 g	13.4	20.7	0.0	*LIND*

Ostrich

Ostrich biltong	25 g	2.5	15.8	0.0	
Ostrich meat (cooked)#	100 g	3.5	25.4	0.0	

Other

Bat, flying (dried)	75 g	35.2	28.7	4.5	
Hare (stewed)#	100 g	8.0	29.9	0.0	
Mopane worm (dried)	50 g	7.3	28.4	0.0	

GREEN FOOD LIST					
Food/product	Portion/ serving size	Fat (g)	Protein (g)	Glycaemic/ net carb (g)	*LIND* (low insulinogenic, nutrient dense
Rabbit (stewed)#	100 g	3.5	33.0	0.4	
Pork					
Bacon, Canadian-style back bacon (grilled)#	100 g	8.4	24.2	1.4	*LIND*
Bacon, cured (pan-fried/grilled)#	50 g	20.9	18.5	0.7	*LIND*
Bacon, cured (pan-fried/grilled)#	75 g	31.4	27.8	1.1	*LIND*
Pork, breast (braised)#	100 g	15.7	26.5	0.0	
Pork, cordon bleu	100 g	19.4	21.7	5.0	
Pork, crackling, no added spices (cooked)#	100 g	49.2	30.5	0.6	
Pork, Kassler rib (grilled)#	100 g	8.4	24.2	1.4	
Pork, leg (roasted)#	100 g	17.6	26.8	0.0	
Pork, loin chop (grilled)#	100 g	13.9	27.3	0.0	
Pork, loin, lean, meat only (braised)#	100 g	7.9	30.2	0.0	
Pork, spare ribs (braised)#	100 g	30.3	29.1	0.0	
Pork, thick rib (braised)#	100 g	15.7	26.5	0.0	
Turkey					
Turkey, bacon (unprepared)	150 g	25.4	23.9	3.5	*LIND*
Turkey, mince (cooked)#	100 g	10.4	27.4	0.0	*LIND*
Turkey, meat & skin (roasted)#	100 g	7.2	28.6	0.1	*LIND*
Turkey, meat only (roasted)#	100 g	3.8	29.1	0.0	*LIND*
Veal (calf)					
Veal, breast (cooked – moist)#	100 g	15.4	23.3	0.0	
Veal, chuck (cooked – moist)#	100 g	8.8	29.3	0.0	
Veal, cordon bleu#	100 g	15.6	22.0	5.3	
Veal, leg (cooked – dry)#	100 g	12.1	27.3	0.0	
Veal, loin (cooked – dry)#	100 g	7.4	25.9	0.0	
Veal, rib (cooked – dry)#	100 g	7.9	25.0	0.0	
Veal, rump (cooked – dry)#	100 g	8.7	27.6	0.0	
Veal, shin (cooked – moist)#	100 g	5.7	31.1	0.0	
Veal, shoulder (cooked – moist)#	100 g	5.8	28.6	0.0	
Fish and seafood					
Anchovy fillets in olive oil	100 g	7.0	20.0	0.0	*LIND*
Anchovy (raw)*	100 g	4.8	20.4	0.0	*LIND*
Angelfish (raw)*	100 g	0.2	20.3	0.0	
Bass, freshwater, mixed species (cooked)#	100 g	4.7	24.2	0.0	
Bass, sea bass, mixed species (cooked)#	100 g	2.6	23.6	0.0	
Bokkom, medium-fat fish (mackerel) (dried, salted)	50 g	5.3	25.0	0.0	
Butterfish, high fat (grilled)#	100 g	11.6	23.0	0.0	
Calamari (raw)*	150 g	2.0	22.56	3.97	
Caviar	100 g	17.9	24.6	3.5	
Cod, Atlantic (cooked)#	100 g	0.9	22.8	0.0	
Cod, Pacific (cooked)#	125 g	0.6	23.4	0.0	
Crab, fresh (cooked)#	125 g	0.9	22.4	0.0	
Fish biltong (cod) (dried, salted)	50 g	1.2	31.4	0.0	
Flatfish, flounder & sole species (cooked)#	150 g	3.6	22.9	0.0	
Haddock, smoked (steamed)#	100 g	1.0	25.2	0.7	
Hake (steamed)#	100 g	2.2	20.0	0.3	
Herring, high fat (grilled)#	100 g	11.6	23.0	0.0	*LIND*
Kingklip (raw)*	150 g	0.4	26.0	0.0	
Kipper, smoked herring (baked)#	100 g	12.4	24.6	1.4	
Lobster, rock/spiny (crayfish) (boiled)#	100 g	1.9	26.4	3.1	

GREEN FOOD LIST					
Food/product	Portion/ serving size	Fat (g)	Protein (g)	Glycaemic/ net carb (g)	*LIND* (low insulinogenic, nutrient dense)
Mackerel, canned in water	100 g	19.5	20.0	1.0	*LIND*
Monkfish (cooked)#	125 g	2.5	23.3	0.0	
Octopus (raw)*	100 g	0.8	12.3	0.0	
Oyster (raw)*	150 g	2.6	6.8	4.1	
Pilchards, canned in brine	100 g	5.4	20.0	0.0	
Prawn (boiled)#	100 g	1.7	22.8	1.5	
Roe (grilled)#	100 g	8.2	28.6	1.9	
Salmon, high fat (steamed)#	100 g	13.0	20.1	0.0	
Salmon, pink excluding bone, canned in water	100 g	0.9	22.4	0.0	
Sardine, canned in oil, drained solids with bone	100 g	11.5	24.6	0.0	*LIND*
Shrimp (boiled)#	100 g	1.7	22.8	1.5	
Snoek (raw)*	100 g	5.2	22.0	<1.0	
Sole (grilled)#	150 g	3.6	22.8	0.0	
Tuna, canned in brine, shredded	100 g	0.4	24.9	0.0	
Tuna, canned in water, drained solids	125 g	1.3	24.3	0.0	
Tuna, fresh, bluefin (raw)*	100 g	4.9	23.3	0.0	
Tuna, fresh, bluefin (cooked)#	100 g	6.3	29.9	0.0	
Tuna, fresh, yellowfin (raw)*	100 g	0.5	24.4	0.0	
Tuna, fresh, skipjack (raw)*	100 g	1.0	22.0	0.0	
Trout, rainbow (grilled)#	100 g	5.8	22.9	0.0	
Trout, rainbow, lightly smoked (raw)*	100 g	6.7	21.3	2.9	
Yellowtail (grilled)#	100 g	6.7	29.7	0.0	
Natural and cured meats and sausages					
Beef, cured, pastrami	1 slice/28 g	1.6	6.1	0.1	
Chorizo, pork & beef	1 link/60 g	23.0	14.5	1.1	*LIND*
Frankfurter, beef & pork	200 g	55.2	23.0	3.4	*LIND*
Salami, beef/pork	100 g	31.7	21.1	0.7	
Sausage, smoked, beef & pork	200 g	57.4	24.0	4.8	
DAIRY					
Cheese					
Cheese, Blaauwkrantz	30 g	9.2	6.5	0.6	
Cheese, blue	30 g	11.4	6.1	1.0	*LIND*
Cheese, Brie	30 g	8.3	6.2	0.2	*LIND*
Cheese, Camembert	30 g	7.3	5.9	0.2	*LIND*
Cheese, Cheddar	30 g	9.7	7.4	0.5	*LIND*
Cheese, Cheddar, mature	30 g	9.7	7.4	1.0	*LIND*
Cheese, Colby	30 g	9.6	7.1	1.0	*LIND*
Cheese, cottage, full fat	30 g	3.3	2.8	1.1	*LIND*
Cheese, cream, full fat	30 g	10.2	1.8	1.2	*LIND*
Cheese, Derby	30 g	10.2	7.3	1.6	
Cheese, Edam	30 g	9.5	7.2	0.1	*LIND*
Cheese, Emmental	30 g	21.0	9.0	0.6	
Cheese, feta	30 g	8.3	5.3	0.4	*LIND*
Cheese, goat, hard type	30 g	10.7	9.2	0.7	*LIND*
Cheese, goat, soft type	30 g	6.3	5.6	0.0	*LIND*
Cheese, Gouda	30 g	9.5	7.2	0.1	*LIND*
Cheese, halloumi	30 g	9.3	7.2	0.0	
Cheese, Leicester	30 g	10.1	7.3	0.0	
Cheese, mozzarella	30 g	6.7	6.7	0.7	*LIND*
Cheese, Parmesan	30 g	7.0	7.1	3.5	*LIND*

GREEN FOOD LIST					
Food/product	Portion/ serving size	Fat (g)	Protein (g)	Glycaemic/ net carb (g)	*LIND* (low insulinogenic, nutrient dense
Cheese, Philadelphia	30 g	10.2	2.2	0.7	
Cheese, ricotta	30 g	3.9	3.4	0.9	*LIND*
Cheese, Roquefort (Blaauwkrantz)	30 g	9.2	6.5	0.6	
Cheese, Swiss	30 g	9.5	7.2	0.1	*LIND*
Cream/milk/yoghurt/non-dairy milk and cream					
Cream					
Cream, coconut, raw (liquid expressed from grated meat)	15 ml	5.2	0.5	0.7	
Cream, crème fraîche	30 g	7.6	1.1	1.2	
Cream, fresh, pouring	15 ml	2.8	0.4	1.0	*LIND*
Cream, fresh, whipping	15 ml	5.8	0.3	0.0	*LIND*
Cream, heavy/double	15 ml	8.7	0.2	0.0	*LIND*
Cream, sour	15 ml	2.9	0.3	0.4	*LIND*
Milk					
Almond milk (not commercial type)	15 ml	0.5	0.3	0.1	
Amasi/sour milk	15 ml	0.6	0.5	0.7	
Buttermilk	15 ml	0.5	0.4	0.6	
Buttermilk, cultured	15 ml	0.4	0.5	0.6	
Coconut milk, raw (liquid expressed from grated meat & water)	15 ml	3.6	0.3	0.5	*LIND*
Cow's milk, full cream	30 ml	1.0	0.9	1.5	
Goat's milk	15 ml	0.6	0.5	0.7	
Kefir, whole milk	100 g	5.0	6.0	6.0	
Yoghurt					
Double-cream yoghurt	100 g	6.0	3.6	7.0	
Full-cream yoghurt	100 g	3.4	3.3	5.0	
Greek full-cream yoghurt	100 g	5.2	5.0	8.0	
FATS AND OILS					
Fats					
Beef tallow	15 ml	15.0	0.0	0.0	
Butter	15 ml	12.4	0.0	0.0	*LIND*
Butter, unsalted	15 ml	12.4	0.0	0.0	*LIND*
Chicken fat	15 ml	15.0	0.0	0.0	
Duck fat	15 ml	15.0	0.0	0.0	
Ghee/clarified butter	15 ml	15.1	0.0	0.0	*LIND*
Lard	15 ml	15.0	0.0	0.0	
Mutton tallow	15 ml	15.0	0.0	0.0	
Oils					
Almond oil	15 ml	13.7	0.0	0.0	
Avocado oil	15 ml	13.6	0.1	0.0	
Coconut oil	15 ml	15.0	0.0	0.0	*LIND*
Coconut oil, organic	15 ml	13.6	0.0	0.0	*LIND*
Cod liver oil/fish oil	15 ml	15.0	0.0	0.0	*LIND*
Macadamia oil	15 ml	13.6	0.0	0.0	
Olive oil	15 ml	15.0	0.0	0.0	*LIND*
Olive oil, extra-virgin	15 ml	13.7	0.0	0.0	*LIND*
Other nut/seed butters					
Almond nut butter	15 ml	8.9	3.8	1.7	
Cocoa butter	15 ml	15.0	0.0	0.0	

GREEN FOOD LIST					
Food/product	Portion/ serving size	Fat (g)	Protein (g)	Glycaemic/ net carb (g)	*LIND* (low insulinogenic, nutrient dense)
Macadamia nut butter	15 ml	12.8	1.2	0.7	
Tahini/sesame butter	15 ml	8.0	3.0	3.0	
FLAVOURING AND CONDIMENTS					
Allspice, ground	5 ml	0.4	0.3	2.5	
Aniseed	5 ml	0.8	0.9	1.8	
Apple cider vinegar (raw, unfiltered)	15 ml	0.0	0.0	0.0	
Bay leaf	5 ml	0.4	0.4	2.4	
Baking powder	5 ml	0.0	0.0	1.2	
Basil, dried	5 ml	0.2	1.2	0.5	
Basil, fresh	1 leaf (0.5 g)	0.0	0.0	0.0	
Basil, fresh, chopped	15 ml (2.65 g)	0.0	0.1	0.1	
Capers, canned, drained	15 ml (8.6 g)	0.1	0.2	0.1	
Caraway seed	5 ml	0.3	0.4	0.3	
Cardamom, ground	5 ml	0.1	0.2	0.8	
Cayenne pepper	5 ml	0.9	0.6	1.5	*LIND*
Celery seed	5 ml	0.5	0.4	0.6	
Chervil, dried	5 ml	0.0	0.1	0.2	
Chillies, powdered	5 ml	0.4	0.4	0.4	
Chives, freeze-dried	5 ml	0.2	1.1	1.9	*LIND*
Cinnamon, ground	5 ml	0.0	0.1	0.7	
Cloves, ground	5 ml	0.3	0.1	0.7	
Cocoa powder	5 ml	1.1	0.9	0.6	
Coriander leaf, dried	5 ml	0.2	1.1	2.1	*LIND*
Coriander leaf, fresh	5 ml	0.0	0.1	0.0	*LIND*
Coriander seed	5 ml	0.3	0.2	0.2	*LIND*
Cumin seed	5 ml	0.9	0.9	0.6	
Curry powder	5 ml	0.7	0.7	0.1	
Dill seed	5 ml	0.3	0.3	0.8	
Dill weed, dried	5 ml	0.0	0.2	0.5	
Dill weed, fresh	5 sprigs (1 g)	0.0	0.03	0.1	
Dill weed, fresh	1 cup sprigs (8.9 g)	0.1	0.3	0.4	
Fennel seed	5 ml whole (2 g)	0.3	0.3	0.3	
Fennel seed	15 ml whole (5.8 g)	0.9	0.9	0.7	
Fenugreek seed	5 ml	0.3	1.2	1.7	
Garam masala	5 ml	0.8	0.8	1.1	
Garlic powder	5 ml	0.0	0.8	3.2	
Garlic, raw	5 ml	0.0	0.3	1.6	
Ginger, ground	5 ml	0.2	0.5	2.9	
Ginger root, fresh	5 ml	0.0	0.1	0.6	
Himalayan crystal pink salt, fine or coarse	5 ml	0.0	0.0	0.0	
Horseradish, prepared	5 ml	0.0	0.1	0.4	
Lemon juice, canned or bottled	5 ml	0.0	0.0	0.3	
Lemon juice, raw, freshly squeezed	5 ml	0.0	0.0	0.3	
Lime juice, canned or bottled (unsweetened)	5 ml	0.0	0.0	0.3	
Lime juice, raw, freshly squeezed	5 ml	0.0	0.0	0.4	
Mace, ground	5 ml	0.6	0.1	0.6	
Marjoram, dried	5 ml	0.0	0.1	0.2	
Mustard seed, ground	5 ml	1.8	1.3	0.8	
Mustard seed, yellow	5 ml	1.8	1.3	0.8	

GREEN FOOD LIST					
Food/product	Portion/ serving size	Fat (g)	Protein (g)	Glycaemic/ net carb (g)	*LIND* (low insulinogenic, nutrient dense
Nutmeg, ground	5 ml	1.8	0.3	1.4	
Origanum, dried	5 ml	0.1	0.2	0.4	
Origanum, dried	1 leaf (1 g)	0.0	0.1	0.3	
Paprika	5 ml	0.6	0.7	1.0	
Parsley, dried	5 ml	0.0	0.1	0.2	
Parsley, fresh	5 ml	0.0	0.2	0.2	*LIND*
Pepper, black	5 ml	0.2	0.5	1.9	
Pepper, red	5 ml	0.3	0.2	0.5	
Pepper, white	5 ml	0.1	0.3	1.1	
Peppermint, fresh	5 ml	0.0	0.2	0.3	
Rosemary, dried	5 ml	0.8	0.2	1.1	*LIND*
Rosemary, fresh	5 ml	0.3	0.2	0.3	
Saffron	5 ml	0.0	0.1	0.5	
Sage, dried	5 ml	0.6	0.5	1.0	
Sage, ground	5 ml	0.1	0.1	0.1	
Salt, table	5 ml	0.0	0.0	0.0	
Salt, table, iodised	5 ml	0.0	0.0	0.0	
Spearmint, dried	5 ml	0.0	0.1	0.2	
Spearmint, fresh	1 leaf (0.15 g)	0.0	0.0	0.0	
Spearmint, fresh	5 ml	0.0	0.2	0.1	
Tabasco sauce	5 ml	0.0	0.1	0.0	
Tarragon, dried	5 ml	0.1	0.4	0.7	
Thyme, dried	5 ml	0.4	0.5	1.3	
Thyme, fresh	5 ml	0.1	0.3	0.5	
Turmeric/borrie, ground	5 ml	0.2	0.5	2.2	
Vanilla extract	5 ml	0.0	0.0	0.5	
Vinegar	5 ml	0.0	0.0	0.0	
Vinegar, balsamic	5 ml	0.0	0.0	0.9	
Vinegar, distilled	5 ml	0.0	0.0	0.0	
Vinegar, red wine	5 ml	0.0	0.0	0.0	
Worcestershire sauce	5 ml	0.0	0.1	0.8	
Yeast, bakers, dried	5 ml	0.1	1.8	0.2	
BEVERAGES					
Coffee and tea					
Coffee, brewed/instant (pure coffee, not canned)	5 ml	0.0	0.0	0.0	
Tea, brewed	100 g	0.0	0.0	0.3	
Tea, green tea, brewed, from bags	1 cup	0.0	0.4	0.0	
Tea, herb, brewed	100 g	0.0	0.0	0.3	
Tea, instant, unsweetened, powder, decaffeinated	10 ml	0.0	0.1	0.3	
Tea, instant, unsweetened, powder, prepared	1 cup	0.0	0.1	0.4	
Tea, rooibos, brewed	100 g	0.0	0.0	0.2	
NUTS, SEEDS AND FLOURS					
Nuts					
Almond, dried, blanched	30 g	15.8	6.4	2.6	*LIND*
Brazil nut, dried, unblanched	30 g	19.9	4.3	1.4	*LIND*
Coconut, desiccated, unsweetened	30 g	19.4	2.1	2.2	*LIND*
Coconut, flesh, raw	30 g	11.7	1.0	0.7	*LIND*
Hazelnut, dried, unblanched	30 g	18.2	4.5	2.1	
Macadamia nut, dried	30 g	22.7	2.4	1.6	*LIND*

Food/product	Portion/ serving size	Fat (g)	Protein (g)	Glycaemic/ net carb (g)	*LIND* (low insulinogenic, nutrient dense)
Pecan nut, dried	30 g	21.6	2.8	1.3	*LIND*
Pine nut	30 g	20.5	4.1	2.8	*LIND*
Pistachio nut, dried	30 g	13.6	6.1	5.2	*LIND*
Walnut, dried	30 g	19.6	4.6	2.1	
Seeds					
Chia seed	10 g	3.1	1.6	4.2	
Coriander seed	5 g	0.9	0.6	0.7	
Flaxseed	5 g	1.7	1.0	0.3	
Linseed	5 g	1.8	0.9	0.2	
Poppy seed	1 g	0.4	0.2	0.0	
Poppy seed	5 g	2.1	0.9	0.5	
Pumpkin seed, whole-roasted	5 g	1.0	0.9	1.8	*LIND*
Sesame seed, dried, hulled	5 g	3.1	1.0	0.0	
Sunflower seed, dried	5 g	2.6	1.0	0.6	*LIND*
Flours					
Almond flour	5 g	2.5	1.1	0.9	
Almond flour	15 g	7.5	3.2	2.8	
Coconut, milled, standard brand	5 g	0.9	0.9	0.9	
Coconut, milled, standard brand	15 g	2.7	2.8	2.8	
Flaxseed/linseed powder	15 ml	1.0	2.9	<1	
Heba (approved by The Noakes Foundation)	5 g	1.1	1.1	0.4	
Heba	15 g	3.3	3.3	1.2	
Psyllium husk	5 g	0.0	0.1	0.2	
Psyllium husk	15 g	0.0	0.2	0.5	
Psyllium husk powder	5 g	0.0	0.0	4.5	
SWEETENERS (not recommended)					
Erythritol granules	5 ml	0.0	0.0	0.0	
Stevia powder	1.5 ml/1.5 g	0.0	0.0	0.0	
Xylitol granules	5 ml	0.0	0.0	0.0	
VEGETABLES AND FRUITS					
Vegetables					
Amadumbe/taro leaves (steamed)#	1 cup	1.0	6.8	5.0	
Amaranth/marog/morogo (boiled)#	1 cup	0.6	4.8	3.0	
Artichoke, globe/French (boiled)#	½ cup	0.4	3.6	4.3	*LIND*
Arugula/salad rocket (raw)*	½ cup	0.9	3.2	2.6	
Asparagus, green (boiled)#	1 cup	0.7	5.7	2.7	
Aubergine/brinjal/eggplant, flesh & skin (boiled)#	½ cup	0.0	0.9	4.0	
Bamboo shoots (raw)*	1 cup	0.7	6.2	2.7	
Broccoli (boiled)#	1 cup	0.7	5.5	3.7	*LIND*
Broccoli (raw)*	½ cup	0.3	4.8	3.9	*LIND*
Brussels sprouts (boiled)#	1 cup	0.2	7.0	5.5	*LIND*
Cabbage (boiled)#	½ cup	0.0	1.3	4.0	
Cabbage (raw)*	½ cup	0.1	1.9	5.4	
Cabbage, Chinese (pe-tsai) (boiled)#	1 cup	0.2	1.8	4.6	
Cabbage, Chinese (pe-tsai) (raw)*	1 cup	0.2	2.2	5.6	
Cabbage, red (boiled)#	½ cup	0.3	1.3	3.3	
Calabash/gourd, white (boiled)#	½ cup	0.0	0.8	3.1	
Capers, canned	1 cup	2.2	6.0	4.2	
Cauliflower (boiled)#	1 cup	0.2	4.2	5.2	

GREEN FOOD LIST

Food/product	Portion/ serving size	Fat (g)	Protein (g)	Glycaemic/ net carb (g)	*LIND* (low insulinogenic, nutrient dense)
Cauliflower (raw)*	½ cup	0.3	2.3	4.3	
Celery (boiled)#	1 cup	0.2	1.2	3.8	
Celery (raw)*	1 cup	0.4	2.4	5.2	
Chives (raw)*	1 cup	1.8	8.2	4.8	
Collards (raw)*	100 g	0.6	3.0	1.4	*LIND*
Collards (boiled, drained)#	1 cup	1.8	6.8	4.2	*LIND*
Cucumber, flesh & skin (raw)*	½ cup	0.1	0.9	2.4	
Cucumber, English, flesh & skin (raw*)	½ cup	0.1	0.9	2.5	
Cucumber, wild (raw)*	½ cup	0.9	1.4	5.6	
Endive (raw)*	100 g	0.2	1.0	1.6	
Fenugreek, leaves (raw)*	100 g	0.2	4.6	4.8	
Gherkins/cucumber, dill, pickled*	100 g	0.3	0.5	1.4	
Green beans (boiled)#	1 cup	0.5	4.5	6.5	
Green beans (raw)*	100 g	0.1	2.1	3.8	
Kale (boiled)#	150 g	0.6	2.9	5.4	*LIND*
Kale (raw)*	100 g	0.9	4.3	5.2	*LIND*
Kohlrabi (boiled)#	100 g	0.1	1.8	5.6	
Kohlrabi (raw)*	100 g	0.1	1.7	2.6	
Leek (boiled)#	100 g	0.2	0.8	6.6	
Lettuce (raw)*	½ cup	0.1	1.1	2.1	
Melon, gemsbok (raw)*	100 g	0.2	1.3	5.0	
Mixed vegetables (cauliflower, carrot, green beans, etc.), frozen (raw)*	100 g	0.3	1.4	3.6	
Mixed vegetables stir-fry (baby marrow, carrot, etc.), frozen (raw)*	100 g	0.2	1.1	4.9	
Mushrooms (boiled)#	½ cup	0.3	2.9	3.4	*LIND*
Mushrooms (raw)*	½ cup	0.3	2.9	3.4	*LIND*
Mushrooms, baby button (raw)*	½ cup	0.9	2.9	0.4	*LIND*
Mushrooms, brown (raw)*	½ cup	0.3	2.9	0.4	*LIND*
Mushrooms, brown, Italian/cremini (raw)*	100 g	0.1	2.5	3.7	*LIND*
Mushrooms, oyster (boiled)#	100 g	0.5	2.2	3.1	*LIND*
Mushrooms, oyster (raw)*	100 g	0.4	3.3	3.8	*LIND*
Mushrooms, portobello (grilled)#	½ cup	0.7	4.1	2.8	*LIND*
Mushrooms, shiitake (raw)*	100 g	0.5	2.2	4.3	*LIND*
Mushrooms, white (raw)*	½ cup	0.4	3.9	2.8	*LIND*
Mushrooms, white (stir-fried)#	½ cup	0.4	4.5	2.8	*LIND*
Mustard greens (raw)*	100 g	0.4	2.9	1.5	*LIND*
Mustard greens (boiled, drained)#	½ cup	0.6	3.2	3.1	*LIND*
Okra (boiled)#	1 cup	0.6	4.8	5.0	
Okra (raw)*	100 g	0.2	1.9	4.3	
Onion (boiled)#	50 g	0.1	0.5	4.4	
Onion (raw)*	50 g	0.1	0.5	4.4	
Onion, pickled, drained solids*	50 g	0.1	0.5	2.4	
Onion, red (raw)*	50 g	0.1	0.5	3.6	
Onion, spring/scallion, includes tops & bulb (raw)*	50 g	1.0	0.9	2.4	
Pepper, chilli (raw)*	100 g	0.5	2.6	4.9	*LIND*
Pepper, hot chilli, green (raw)*	50 g	0.1	1.0	4.0	*LIND*
Pepper, hot chilli, red (raw)*	50 g	0.2	0.9	3.7	*LIND*
Pepper, jalapeño (raw)*	100 g	0.4	0.9	3.7	*LIND*

GREEN FOOD LIST

Food/product	Portion/ serving size	Fat (g)	Protein (g)	Glycaemic/ net carb (g)	*LIND* (low insulinogenic, nutrient dense)
Pepper, sweet, green (boiled)#	50 g	0.1	0.7	2.4	*LIND*
Pepper, sweet, green (raw)*	50 g	0.1	0.5	1.6	*LIND*
Pepper, sweet, red (boiled)#	50 g	0.1	0.5	2.8	*LIND*
Pepper, sweet, red (raw)*	50 g	0.2	0.5	2.0	*LIND*
Pepper, sweet, yellow (raw)*	50 g	0.1	0.5	2.7	*LIND*
Pumpkin (boiled)#	½ cup	0.1	0.9	3.6	
Radish (raw)*	100 g	0.1	0.7	1.8	
Ratatouille*	100 g	4.6	1.1	4.1	
Sauerkraut, canned, solids & liquids	100 g	0.1	0.9	1.4	
Seaweed, spirulina (raw)*	5 g	0.0	0.3	0.1	
Seaweed, spirulina, dried	15 ml	0.5	4.0	1.4	
Seaweed, wakame (raw)*	60 g	0.4	1.8	5.2	
Sou-sou/chayote (boiled)#	1 cup	0.2	1.8	6.6	
Sou-sou/chayote (raw)*	100 g	0.1	0.7	2.6	
Spinach, small-leaved (boiled)#	1 cup	0.8	7.6	3.6	*LIND*
Spinach, small-leaved (raw)*	½ cup	0.5	3.6	1.8	*LIND*
Spinach, Swiss chard (boiled)#	1 cup	0.7	6.7	5.0	*LIND*
Spinach, Swiss chard (raw)*	½ cup	0.3	3.4	2.0	*LIND*
Spring onion/scallion, includes tops & bulb, chopped*	1 cup	0.2	1.8	4.7	
Spring onion/scallion, includes tops & bulb*	1 large (25 g)	0.1	0.5	1.2	
Squash, baby marrow/courgette/zucchini (boiled)#	1 cup	0.2	3.8	3.0	
Squash, gem, flesh only (boiled)#	½ cup	0.1	0.6	4.4	
Squash, hubbard (boiled)#	100 g	0.1	0.7	5.6	
Squash, marrow (boiled)#	½ cup	0.0	0.1	2.1	
Squash, patty pan (boiled)#	½ cup	0.3	1.3	1.8	
Squash, table queen (boiled)#	50 g	0.1	0.5	3.5	
Sugarsnap peas*	100 g	0.1	28.0	5.3	
Tomato (boiled)#	½ cup	0.4	1.5	5.0	
Tomato (raw)*	½ cup	0.3	1.1	3.6	
Tomato & onion, canned	50 g	0.0	0.7	3.8	
Tomato & onion, stewed, no sugar#	100 g	0.3	1.1	5.2	
Tomato, cocktail (raw)*	½ cup	0.6	1.3	2.9	
Tomato paste	5 g	0.0	0.2	0.7	
Tomato purée	5 g	0.0	0.1	0.5	
Tomato, whole peeled/chopped, canned	100 g	0.1	0.8	3.4	
Truffle, Kalahari (raw)*	100 g	3.5	4.1	0.8	
Turnip (boiled)#	½ cup	0.1	0.9	3.9	*LIND*
Waterblommetjies (boiled)#	1 cup	0.0	1.8	5.2	
Waterblommetjies, canned	100 g	0.0	0.5	1.6	
Watercress (raw)*	½ cup	0.1	2.9	1.0	
Wild rocket	½ cup	0.3	4.4	0.0	
Wild rocket	1 cup	0.6	8.8	0.0	
Fruits					
Avocado, peeled (raw)*	50 g	11.8	0.9	1.0	*LIND*
Olive, canned, drained, pitted*	50 g	5.4	0.4	1.6	*LIND*
Olive, mixed in brine*	35 g	3.8	0.3	3.1	*LIND*

ORANGE FOOD LIST

Food/product	Portion/ serving size	Fat (g)	Protein (g)	Glycaemic/ net carb (g)
REF: * raw weight / # cooked weight. If you are going to eat the food raw, weigh It and work on raw weight only; if you are going to cook the food, only weigh the food once cooked and work on cooked values.				
FRUITS				
Apple, average (raw)*	50 g	0.1	0.1	6.5
Apple, average, without skin (raw)*	50 g	0.1	0.2	5.8
Apple, Golden Delicious (raw)*	50 g	0.0	0.1	6.8
Apple, Granny Smith (raw)*	50 g	0.0	0.1	6.5
Apple, Starking (raw)*	50 g	0.1	0.1	7.0
Apricot (raw)*	100 g	0.1	0.8	6.5
Banana, peeled (raw)*	50 g	0.2	0.7	9.4
Blackberries (raw)*	100 g	0.5	1.4	4.3
Blueberries (raw)*	50 g	0.2	0.4	6.1
Cherries (raw)*	50 g	0.1	0.6	6.7
Clementines (raw)*	50 g	0.1	0.4	5.2
Cranberries (raw)*	50 g	0.1	0.2	3.8
Figs (raw)*	50 g	0.5	0.6	6.8
Gooseberries, Cape (raw)*	100 g	0.7	1.9	6.0
Granadilla, peeled (raw)*	50 g	0.2	1.1	6.5
Grape, average (raw)*	50 g	0.1	0.4	7.4
Grape, sultana (raw)*	50 g	0.1	0.4	7.7
Grapefruit, peeled (raw)*	100 g	0.1	0.7	6.9
Guava, peeled (raw)*	100 g	0.3	0.8	7.7
Kiwifruit, peeled (raw)*	50 g	0.3	0.5	6.5
Kumquat (raw)*	50 g	0.5	1.0	4.7
Lemon, peeled (raw)*	100 g	0.2	0.7	7.0
Lime, peeled (raw)*	100 g	0.2	0.7	7.7
Litchi, peeled (raw)*	50 g	0.1	0.4	8.6
Loquat (raw)*	50 g	0.1	0.2	5.2
Mango, peeled (raw)*	50 g	0.1	0.3	7.65
Marula, peeled (raw)*	50 g	0.2	0.3	6.1
Medlar, wild (raw)*	50 g	0.0	0.7	11.1
Melon, cantaloupe (raw)*	100 g	0.2	0.8	7.3
Melon, green flesh, peeled (raw)*	50 g	0.1	0.4	4.5
Melon, honeydew (raw)*	50 g	0.1	0.3	4.2
Melon, orange flesh, peeled (raw)*	50 g	0.1	0.4	4.1
Melon, tsama (raw)*	50 g	0.1	0.3	4.2
Melon, wild (raw)*	100 g	0.2	1.4	4.0
Minneola, peeled (raw)*	50 g	0.1	0.4	4.7
Mulberries (raw)*	50 g	0.2	0.7	4.1
Naartjie/tangerine, peeled (raw)*	50 g	0.1	0.5	5.0
Nectarine (raw)*	50 g	0.1	0.4	5.2
Num-num (raw)*	100 g	1.2	0.7	6.5
Orange, peeled (raw)*	50 g	0.1	0.4	4.6
Papaya (raw)*	50 g	0.2	0.3	4.6
Pawpaw, peeled (raw)*	50 g	0.1	0.2	4.3
Peach (raw)*	50 g	0.1	0.4	4.3
Peach, yellow cling (raw)*	50 g	0.1	0.4	5.5
Pear (raw)*	50 g	0.1	0.2	7.2
Persimmon, peeled (raw)*	50 g	0.1	0.3	7.5
Pineapple, peeled (raw)*	50 g	0.1	0.2	6.1

ORANGE FOOD LIST				
Food/product	Portion/ serving size	Fat (g)	Protein (g)	Glycaemic/ net carb (g)
Plum (raw)*	50 g	0.1	0.4	5.5
Plum, Natal, peeled (raw)*	50 g	0.6	0.3	5.1
Pomegranate, peeled (raw)*	50 g	0.6	0.9	7.4
Prickly pear, peeled (raw)*	50 g	0.2	0.5	5.3
Prune (raw)*	50 g	0.1	0.4	6.5
Quince, peeled (raw)*	50 g	0.1	0.2	6.7
Raspberries (raw)*	100 g	0.7	1.2	5.4
Rhubarb, stems (raw)*	100 g	0.2	0.9	2.7
Starfruit/carambola (raw)*	100 g	0.3	1.0	3.9
Strawberries (raw)*	100 g	0.3	0.7	6.0
Watermelon, peeled (raw)*	100 g	0.1	0.9	5.9
Youngberries (raw)*	100 g	0.5	1.4	4.3
NUTS				
Betel nut	30 g	3.2	1.8	16.1
Cashew nut, dry-roasted, unsalted	30 g	13.9	4.6	8.9
Chestnut, fresh, peeled	30 g	0.4	0.5	13.3
NUT BUTTER				
Cashew nut butter	15 g	7.0	2.3	4.7
SWEETENERS				
Honey	5 g	0.0	0.0	4.0
VEGETABLES				
Artichoke, Jerusalem (boiled)#	100 g	0.0	1.8	14.3
Artichoke, Jerusalem (raw)*	100 g	0.0	2.0	15.8
Beetroot (cooked)#	100 g	0.18	1.68	7.96
Carrot, flesh and skin (boiled)#	100 g	0.1	0.9	5.3
Carrot, flesh and skin (raw)*	100 g	0.0	0.9	6.4
Leek (raw)*	100 g	0.3	1.5	12.4
Parsnip (cooked)#	100 g	0.3	1.32	13.01
Onion, dehydrated (boiled)#	50 g	0.1	0.7	6.1
Squash, butternut (boiled)#	100 g	0.1	1.5	10.2
Sweet potato, orange-fleshed (baked with skin – flesh only)#	100 g	0.2	2.0	17.4
Sweet potato, white-fleshed (boiled without skin)#	100 g	0.1	1.0	15.1
Tomato, sun-dried	25 g	0.8	3.5	10.9
PROTEINS				
Abalone (fried)#	125 g	8.5	24.5	14.6
Mussel, black/blue (boiled)#	100 g	4.5	23.8	7.4
Perlemoen (fried)#	125 g	8.5	24.5	14.6
Snail/whelk (boiled)#	75 g	0.6	35.8	11.6

RED FOOD LIST

All processed foods will be RED and will contain more than two ingredients that you will find hard to pronounce.

BAKED OR COOKED PRODUCTS EITHER COMMERCIAL/BAKERY OR HOMEMADE

Breads, rolls, etc.

All commercial breads, including retail bakery and health-shop types

All varieties of low-carb, sugar-free, diabetic-friendly or gluten-free breads that contain wheat flour,
artificial sweeteners and other strange ingredients, e.g. white, brown, rye and seed breads,
buns, rolls, wraps, rotis, garlic bread, ciabatta, French loaf, paninis, pies, etc.

Bakery sweet treats, etc.

All commercially baked sweet confectionary, including retail bakery and health-shop types

E.g. tarts, cakes, biscuits, rusks, muffins, scones, pastries, etc.

Grains

E.g. amaranth, barley, oats, quinoa, rye, teff, wheat, etc.

Cereals and breakfast porridge

All commercial cereals, including ones that need to be cooked and instant cereals

E.g. granola (a common ingredient used is oats), bran, kids' cereals, maize/mealie pap, Weet-Bix, etc.

Flours, wheat and starch

All products containing any of these ingredients

Atta (chapati flour)

Barley (flakes, flour, pearl)

Brans

Breaded or battered foods

Breading, bread stuffing, bread flour

Buckwheat

Bulgur

Cake flour

Chickpea flour

Cornflour

Durum (type of wheat)

Einkorn (type of wheat)

Emmer (type of wheat)

Farina

Farro/faro (also known as spelt or dinkel)

Fu (a dried gluten product made from wheat and used in some Asian dishes)

Graham flour

Hydrolysed wheat protein

Kamut (type of wheat)

Malt, malt extract, malt syrup, malt flavouring

Matzo, matzo meal

Millet flour

Modified wheat starch

Oatmeal, oat bran, oat flour, whole oats

Potato starch

Rice flour

Rye bread and flour

Seitan (a meat-like food derived from wheat gluten used in many vegetarian dishes)

Semolina

Spelt (type of wheat also known as farro, faro or dinkel)

Sorghum

Soy flour

Triticale

Wheat bran

Wheat flour, e.g. brown-bread wheat flour/cake wheat flour/self-raising wheat flour

RED FOOD LIST
Wheat germ
Wheat starch
Sides like rice, pasta, etc.
All commercial rices, pastas, etc. including homemade flour pastas
e.g. rice (all types), beans (dried), pasta (all types), barley, couscous, lentils, polenta, spelt, split peas, stampkoring, samp and beans, etc.
BEVERAGES
Alcohol
All varieties, including those claiming to be 'lite'
Beers
Ciders
Dessert wines, such as port
Liqueurs
Shooters
Fizzy drinks
All commercial and homemade (Soda Stream) versions, including 'lite', 'zero' or 'diet' versions
e.g. diet drinks, energy drinks, fizzy drinks, etc.
Fruit drinks
All commercial and homemade drinks, including 'low-calorie' or 'diet' versions
'Aanmaak-koeldrank', juice and cordials (vegetable and fruit)
Other drinks
Canned coffee – generally containing other ingredients like dextrins, maltose, dextrose, etc.
Tea with added artificial ingredients
CANNED/BOTTLED/BOXED PRODUCTS
E.g. biscuit pre-mixes, bread spreads, jellies, cake and muffin pre-mixes, dessert boxes, thickening agents such as gravy powder, maize starch or stock cubes, soup packets (powdered and fresh), packet sauces, spices and herbs that contain sugar, e.g. mixed spices (BBQ, etc.), etc.
DAIRY AND DAIRY-RELATED PRODUCTS
Cheese
All commercial cheeses containing more than two or three ingredients on the label
Cheese spreads
Processed cheese – usually packaged as single slices/small blocks/triangles/big soft blocks/flavoured
Tub cheese – low-fat or reduced-fat or flavoured
Cream
All commercial powdered or canned creams
Canned cream (dessert/whipping)
Coffee creamer (powder)
Milk
All low-fat/fat-free/reduced-fat/powdered milks
% low-fat milk
Commercial almond milk
Condensed milk
Custard
Fat-free milk
Flavoured yoghurt
Ice cream
Low-fat milk
Low-fat yoghurt
Powdered milk such as almond/soy, etc.
Puddings
Rice milk
Soy milk

RED FOOD LIST
FATS AND OILS
Fats
All commercial fat spreads/margarines, etc.

Block margarine
Flavoured butters, e.g. garlic or herbs
Margarine

Oils and sauces
All oils that cannot withstand heat, and sauces

Barbecue sauce
Blended cooking oils
Canola (rapeseed) oil
Chilli sauce
Chutney
Cook-in- sauces – bottle and packet variety
Corn oil
Cottonseed (hydrogenated)
Cottonseed oil
Grapeseed oil
Hydrogenated or partially hydrogenated oils including margarine, vegetable oils, vegetable fats, etc.
Marinades
Mayonnaise
Mustard sauce
Palm (hydrogenated)
Pasta sauces – bottle and packet variety
Peanut oil
Peri-peri sauce
Safflower (>70% linoleic)
Safflower (high oleic)
Salad creams
Salad dressings
Seed oils and olive-oil blends – be careful of these, as they catch Banters out!
Soy sauces
Soybean (hydrogenated)
Soybean oil
Steakhouse sauces
Sunflower (<60% linoleic)
Sunflower (>70% oleic)
Sweet sauces, e.g. chocolate sauce
Thousand Island sauces
Tomato sauce

GENERAL
Fast food and takeaways

Burgers
Crumbed/battered chicken, fish or meat
Desserts
Fries
Hotdogs/foot-longs
Pizzas
Wraps
Others not mentioned on the list

So-called health or Banting products
Be especially aware of these so-called health products: they are commonly found in health shops and the health aisles of supermarkets

RED FOOD LIST

Agave nectar

Banting friendly – watch out for shakes or products claiming to be Banting friendly

Blackstrap molasses

Bread pre-mixes

Cake flour

Chocolate almond butter

Coconut milk powder/almond milk powder

Gluten-free flour mixes/self-raising flour/cake and biscuit mixes

Just protein (soy) whey proteins

Polenta

Puffed brown rice

Quinoa (red and white mixed)

Rice cakes/crackers

Rice milk powder

Rolled oats (gluten free)

Slimming shakes – any kind

Soy lecithin granules

Soy milk powder

Soy mince (organic)

Soy sauces

Tamari, organic

Wheat germ

Others not mentioned on the list

MEAT AND MEAT-RELATED PRODUCTS

Canned meats

Corned meat

Meatballs

Pilchards in tomato sauce

Sardines in tomato sauce

Tuna in vegetable oil

Viennas in brine, etc.

Others not mentioned on the list

Frozen meats

Beef patties

Breast steaks

Chicken steaklets

Chickaroos

Crumbed chicken burger patties

Crumbed chicken fingers

Crumbed fish

Crumbed nuggets

Fish bakes

Fish fingers

Meal boxes

Meat pies

Meat-free sausages (soy), etc.

Ready-made meals

Snackaroos

Others not mentioned on the list

Processed, cured and marinated meats

Any meat that has been cured with sugar and/or marinated meats with added ingredients

Any unfermented soy, e.g. vegetarian 'protein' found in ready-made meals, patties, etc.

RED FOOD LIST

Boerewors that contains more than two ingredients (they generally have an ingredient label)
Cold processed meats, e.g. sandwich ham/ham/chicken/beef, etc. generally found at the deli
Crumbed/battered meat, e.g. crumbed chicken or hamburger patties or crumbed fish fingers (fresh variety)
Frankfurters/processed salami
Liver spreads or pâtés – usually sealed in tubes
Luncheon meats
Marinated chops like lamb, pork, beef, etc.
Marinated ribs
Meat with spices
Other types of sausages that contain more than two ingredients (they generally have an ingredient label)
Polonies
Rookworst, debrecener, etc.
Viennas – chicken, plain and diet variety

NUTS/DRIED FRUIT/SWEETS, ETC.

Nuts and dried fruit

All varieties of dried fruits
Chocolate-coated nuts
Nuts coated in different spices
Nuts mixed with dried fruits
Sugar-coated nuts

Sweets and salty snacks

Choc-chip biscuits	All types of chocolates	All types of chips
Lemon Creams	All types of sweets	All types of maize snacks
Marie biscuits	Chewing gum – even those that claim to be sugar free	Corn thins
Rusks	Gummy sweets	Cracker breads
Shortbread	Mallows	Flavoured crackers
Sweet biscuits	Popcorn	Provitas
Tennis biscuits	Pretzels	Rice cakes
Wafers	Toffees	Salticrax

STARCHY VEGETABLES AND VEGETABLE-RELATED PRODUCTS

Fresh starchy vegetables, fruits and legumes

Vegetables	Fruits	Legumes
Bean sprouts, alfalfa	Dates	*Beans*
Bean sprouts, lentils		Adzuki beans
Bean sprouts, mung		Anasazi beans
Corn (mealies)		Black beans
Potatoes (all kinds)		Fava beans
		Garbanzo beans (chickpeas)
		Kidney beans
		Lima beans
		Soybeans
		Nuts
		Carob nuts
		Peanuts
		Soy nuts
		Peas
		Black-eyed peas
		Green peas
		Snap peas

RED FOOD LIST		
		Snow peas
		Split peas
Canned/bottled vegetables		
Beans in a bottle, can or box – borlotti, baked, red kidney, butter, etc.		
Beetroot – bottle and box varieties		
Boxed salads of any kind		
Carrots in brine		
Chickpeas		
Cream-style sweetcorn		
Garden peas		
Lentils		
Mushrooms in brine		
Standard corn (pitted)		
Others not mentioned on the list		
Frozen vegetables		
Mixed varieties of peas and sweetcorn		
Peas		
Potato chips		
Sweetcorn		
Vegetables in sauces, e.g. creamed spinach		
SWEETENERS		
All single-packaged or bottled sugars and products that contain those sugars and related products included in the Ingredients List		

YELLOW FOOD LIST

Food/product	Portion/serving size	Fat (g)	Protein (g)	Glycaemic/net carb (g)
BANTING FRIENDLY				
Shop friendly				
Grain-free crackers (Life Bake)	8 g	1	2	0
Grain-free granola (Life Bake)	40 g	9	8	1
Grain-free toast (Life Bake)	25 g	3	5	1
Low-carb rusks (The Gluten Free Gurus)	1 rusk	9	3	2

Note: If you are not sure if the product is Banting friendly, always refer to the Ingredients List and if the product contains any of the warning ingredients, then you know it's a false Banting product.

BEVERAGES				
Coconut water	100 ml	0	<0.20	6
Alcohol				

Note: Only occasionally. During weight-loss stage, alcohol is NOT recommended!

Food/product	Portion/serving size	Fat (g)	Protein (g)	Glycaemic/net carb (g)
Spirit, brandy (alc 43% v/v; 33% w/w)	Single (25 ml)	0	0	0
Spirit, cane (alc 43% v/v; 33% w/w)	Single (25 ml)	0	0	0
Spirit, gin (alc 43% v/v; 33% w/w)	Single (25 ml)	0	0	0
Spirit, rum (alc 43% v/v; 33% w/w)	Single (25 ml)	0	0	0
Spirit, vodka (alc 43% v/v; 33% w/w)	Single (25 ml)	0	0	0
Spirit, whisky (alc 43% v/v; 33% w/w)	Single (25 ml)	0	0	0
Wine, red dry (alc 12% v/v; 10% w/w)	100 ml standard serve	0	0	3
Wine, red semi-sweet (alc 12% v/v; 10% w/w)	100 ml standard serve	0	0	3
Wine, red sparkling (alc 12% v/v; 10% w/w)	150 ml standard serve	0	0	5
Wine, rosé dry (alc 12% v/v; 10% w/w)	100 ml standard serve	0	0	3
Wine, rosé semi-sweet (alc 12% v/v; 10% w/w)	100 ml standard serve	0	0	3
Wine, rosé sparkling (alc 12% v/v; 10% w/w)	150 ml standard serve	0	0	5
Wine, white dry (alc 12% v/v; 10% w/w)	100 ml standard serve	0	0	3
Wine, white semi-sweet (alc 12% v/v; 10% w/w)	100 ml standard serve	0	0	3
Wine, white sparkling (alc 12% v/v; 10% w/w)	150 ml standard serve	0	0	5
OTHER				
Sweet treats				

Note: Only occasionally. Once every four to six weeks is fine.

Food/product	Portion/serving size	Fat (g)	Protein (g)	Glycaemic/net carb (g)
Lindt Excellence 85% Cocoa chocolate bar (may contain traces of soy lecithin)	20 g (2 squares)	1	2	4
Lindt Excellence 90% Dark chocolate bar (may contain traces of soy lecithin)	20 g (2 squares)	11	2	3

INGREDIENTS LIST		
Please take note: If you look at a label and one of the ingredients is a YES, but the rest are NO, then it means the product is a NO! If all the ingredients in the product are YES, then this makes the product a YES!		
INGREDIENT NAME	YES	NO
SOY AND RELATED PRODUCTS		
Dark soy sauce		NO
Dietary soy protein		NO
Flavonoids		NO
Fortified soymilk		NO
Hydrolysed soy protein		NO
Hydrolysed vegetable protein		NO
Isoflavonoid		NO
Isoflavones		NO
Legume		NO
Soya		NO
Soybean		NO
Soybean-barley paste		NO
Soybean oil		NO
Soy concentrates		NO
Soy fibre		NO
Soy flour		NO
Soy food		NO
Soy isoflavones		NO
Soy isolates		NO
Soy lecithin		NO
Soy milk		NO
Soy nuts		NO
Soy oil		NO
Soy phosphatidylcholine complex (IdB 1016)		NO
Soy phosphatidylinositol (PI)		NO
Soy product		NO
Soy protein		NO
Soy protein isolate		NO
Soy saponins		NO
Soy sauce		NO
Textured vegetable protein		NO
Tofu		NO
Vegetable oil		NO
Yuba		NO
SUGAR AND RELATED PRODUCTS		
Advantame		NO
Agave syrup		NO
Alitame		NO
Acesulfame potassium (acesulfame-K)		NO
Aspartame		NO
Aspartame-acesulfame salt		NO
Barbados sugar		NO
Barley malt		NO
Beet sugar		NO
Blackstrap molasses		NO
Bizzein		NO
Brown sugar		NO
Brown rice syrup		NO

INGREDIENTS LIST		
Please take note: If you look at a label and one of the ingredients is a YES, but the rest are NO, then it means the product is a NO! If all the ingredients in the product are YES, then this makes the product a YES!		
INGREDIENT NAME	**YES**	**NO**
Buttered sugar		NO
Buttered syrup		NO
Cane juice		NO
Cane-juice crystals		NO
Cane sugar		NO
Castor sugar		NO
Caramel		NO
Carob syrup		NO
Coconut sugar		NO
Confectioner's sugar		NO
Concentrate		NO
Corn sweetener		NO
Corn syrup		NO
Corn-syrup solids		NO
Curculin		NO
Crystal fructose		NO
Cyclamates		NO
Cyclamic acid		NO
Date sugar		NO
Demerara sugar		NO
Dextran		NO
Dextrose		NO
Diastatic malt		NO
Diastase		NO
Erythritol	YES	
Ethyl maltol		NO
Evaporated cane juice		NO
Florida crystals		NO
Fructose		NO
Fruit juice		NO
Fruit-juice concentrate		NO
Galactose		NO
Glucose		NO
Glucose solids		NO
Glucose syrup		NO
Glucin		NO
Glycerin		NO
Glycerol		NO
Glycyrrhizin		NO
Golden sugar		NO
Golden syrup		NO
Grape sugar		NO
HFCS (high-fructose corn syrup)		NO
Honey	YES	
Hydrogenated starch hydrolysates		NO
Icing sugar		NO
Inulin		NO
Intense		NO
Invert sugar		NO

Please take note: If you look at a label and one of the ingredients is a YES, but the rest are NO, then it means the product is a NO! If all the ingredients in the product are YES, then this makes the product a YES!

INGREDIENT NAME	YES	NO
vert syrup		NO
omalt		NO
ctitol		NO
ctose	YES	
abinlin		NO
alt sugar		NO
alt syrup		NO
altitol		NO
altodextrin		NO
alto-oligosaccharide		NO
altose		NO
annitol		NO
aple syrup		NO
raculin		NO
ogroside mix		NO
olasses		NO
olasses syrup		NO
onatin		NO
onellin		NO
uscovado sugar		NO
eohesperidin dihydrochalcone		NO
eotame		NO
at syrup		NO
ganic raw sugar		NO
sladin		NO
ntadin		NO
w sugar		NO
efiner's syrup		NO
ce bran syrup		NO
ce malt syrup		NO
ce syrup		NO
accharin		NO
alt of aspartame-acesulfame		NO
odium cyclamate		NO
orbitol		NO
orghum syrup		NO
evia	YES	
cralose		NO
crose		NO
gar		NO
rup		NO
ple sugar		NO
gatose		NO
pioca syrup		NO
aumatin		NO
acle		NO
binado sugar		NO
itol	YES	
low sugar		NO

Further information

Slender Slim 4 U is the first group of slimming clinics in South Africa that specialises in low-carb and healthy high fats, commonly known in South Africa as the Banting lifestyle. At Slender Slim 4 U we teach you how to make a complete lifestyle change simply by changing the way you eat. Slender Slim 4 U does not promote diet pills, shakes or restricted calorie/starvation diets – only good-old, clean eating. Sign up for one of our courses or make an appointment for a consultation with one of our clinic consultants at **www.slenderslim4u.co.za** or at **info@slenderslim4u.co.za**.

The Noakes Foundation was founded in 2012 by Prof. Tim Noakes in response to the critical need for robust research into nutrition. The foundation is a non-profit organisation founded for public benefit that aims to advance medical science's understanding of the benefits of a low-carbohydrate, healthy, high-fat (LCHF) diet by providing evidence-based information on optimum nutrition. The foundation's key goal is to change the way South Africa, and hopefully the world, thinks about food and nutrition. The obesity and type 2 diabetes epidemics are set to cripple global health care within the next 10 years. Something needs to be done before this happens – The Noakes Foundation is taking action.

Eat Better South Africa! was established when The Noakes Foundation realised that the poorest communities around South Africa, whose diet consists mainly of maize and maize products, were unaware of the dangers of excessive sugar and carbohydrate consumption. This has resulted in an unprecedented increase in cases of obesity, type 2 diabetes and other metabolic syndromes. In response to this crisis, The Noakes Foundation team established Eat Better South Africa! (EBSA), a community-outreach branch of the foundation. EBSA is a programme aimed at educating people from lower-income areas, teaching them to get better by eating better. Men and women from these communities sign up to a six-week course where they learn about the benefits of a low-carb, healthy high-fat diet and are assisted in making better food choices through nutritional education, meal and budget planning, and general nutritional awareness.